The Burnout Workbook

Published in the United States by Clarkson Potter/Publishers, an imprint of Random House, a division of Penguin Random House LLC, New York.

ClarksonPotter.com
RandomHouseBooks.com

CLARKSON POTTER is a trademark and POTTER with colophon is a registered trademark of Penguin Random House LLC.

Select material originally appeared in *Burnout: The Secret to Unlocking the Stress Cycle* by Emily Nagoski and Amelia Nagoski, published by Ballantine Books, an imprint of Random House, a division of Penguin Random House LLC, New York, in 2019. Copyright © 2019 by Emily Nagoski, PhD, and Amelia Nagoski, DMA.

Stress Response Cycle comic on page 18, copyright © 2021 by Erika Moen Comics and Illustration, LLC. All rights reserved. Used with permission.

Library of Congress Cataloging-in-Publication Data has been applied for.

ISBN 978-0-593-57837-7

Printed in the USA

Editor: Andrea Bussell

Editorial Assistant: Darian Keels

Designer: Laura Palese

Production Editor: Joyce Wong

Production Manager: Jessica Heim

Copy Editor: Alison Hagge

Marketer: Chloe Aryeh

Workbook and cover design by Danielle Deschenes

2nd Printing

First Edition

The Burnout Workbook

Advice and Exercises to Help You
Unlock the Stress Cycle

Emily Nagoski, PhD, and Amelia Nagoski, DMA

CLARKSON POTTER/PUBLISHERS
NEW YORK

INTRODUCTION

Welcome! The fact that you're reading this probably means you have hope that you can feel better, even if you're feeling overwhelmed and exhausted. And you're right! You **can** feel better. This workbook will show you how.

This workbook grew out of *Burnout: The Secret to Unlocking the Stress Cycle*, our bestselling book about stress, which surveys the ways women exprience being overwhelmed, complete with all the receipts—stories, cultural context, and academic citations from many sciences that detail the problem—so the solutions make sense. The book explains both **how** to feel better and **why** these strategies work when so much mainstream advice for managing stress fails. It was the book Amelia needed when burnout put her in the hospital twice. Since the book came out, we've learned that lots of readers are looking for help **right now**—they just need results ASAP, and the receipts are optional.

Some of the exercises in this workbook will help you right away, some will become strategies you'll use in moments of stress, and some may require practice and time before you start to see how helpful they are. If a certain exercise doesn't seem to click for you, don't worry. That's normal. Not everything will work for everyone. But everyone will find something that helps.

You're Striving to Find Peace. Will This Workbook Give You That?

A lot of folks we've talked to have the goal of reaching a state of peace and staying there. But the body is not built to be only at peace. We're built to oscillate from peace to stress, then return to peace, and back again.

The goal of this workbook is *wellness*. **Wellness is not a state of mind or a state of being. Wellness is a state of action.** It's the freedom to move through all cycles of being human: from effort to rest and back, from autonomy to connection and back, from sleeping to waking, from eating to digesting, from inhaling to exhaling, etc. Burnout happens when we get stuck. These pages will help you notice when you get stuck and show you what you can do to get unstuck.

How to Use This Workbook . . .

Ruin it! Write all over it. Tear things out and stuff them in your planner. Use pens and highlighters, crayons and markers. Circle stuff. Dog-ear pages. Shove it in your bag, carry it everywhere, beat it to hell. The more you interact with it and make it your own, the more you'll learn. Think of this workbook like a lime. You want to use every part—the juice, the zest, and the peel. When you're done, what's left should be a pile of nearly unrecognizable mess. If in the end it still looks like a lime, you haven't squeezed out everything that it has to offer.

Go in order . . . ish. The book is designed to be read from beginning to end. Exercises and information are cumulative, so they will be most effective if you do them in order. That said, if there's something you know you need help with right now (for example, sleep), go ahead and skip straight to that topic. The exercises will still work independently.

Practice nonjudgment. There's an appendix with detailed instructions on mindful nonjudgment, but the short version is this: *Nonjudgment* just means noticing that your brain has flooded your attention with thoughts about how good or bad a thing is, which may not always be relevant, and can be distracting. Set aside thoughts of liking or disliking, and keep your attention on the task at hand.

Don't do anything you don't want to do. There are a wide variety of exercises that use as many senses and ways of thinking as we could manage. In general, if you find an exercise that works for you, great! It's most effective to focus on the ones that use your strengths. And if there's something that doesn't work, also great! It's useful to know what doesn't help. If you're avoiding something because it brings up difficult feelings, we strongly encourage you to find a friend or therapist to work with you.

Spend time on things, but not too much. Assess how much time you're comfortable spending on each exercise. Some will be quick and easy for you, others you may want to spend more time reflecting on. We've provided durations as broad suggestions—if you find yourself spending way less time on an exercise than is suggested, you may not be getting as much out of it as you could. Or if you're spending way more time on an exercise than is suggested, you might want to move on to something else, then come back to it later. They really are just suggestions; no one is watching or timing you. They're meant to give you an idea of what we intended, so you can benefit as much as possible from the work you do.

How These Pages Are Organized . . .

This workbook focuses on managing stress, the cycle that happens in your body. We'll talk a little about managing the things that cause us stress, but our goal is to make you an expert in using your internal resources, and recognizing the ways external social forces interfere with your well-being. Because that expertise will prepare you to deal with *any* problem. We've divided the workbook into three parts.

Part 1: What You Take with You

In the *Star Wars* movie *Episode V: The Empire Strikes Back*, Luke Skywalker sees an evil cave. Looking toward the entrance in dread, he asks his teacher, Yoda, "What's in there?" Yoda answers, "Only what you take with you."

Once you know what you're taking with you, you'll be ready to face the scary stuff. **Part 1 walks you through three internal resources you can rely on to feel better right away:**

1. The stress response cycle

2. The Monitor, or the brain mechanism that controls the emotion of frustration

3. Meaning in life. "Meaning" is often misunderstood as the thing we'll find at the end of the tunnel, but it's not. It's why we go through the tunnel, regardless of what we find on the other end.

More on these later.

Part 2: The Real Enemy

The title of this section is a reference to *The Hunger Games*, in which young Katniss Everdeen is forced into a "game" organized by a dystopian sci-fi government, wherein she must kill other children. Her mentor tells her, "Remember who the real enemy is." It's not the people the government wants her to kill, who are also trying to kill her. The real enemy is the system that set up the game in the first place.

This section is about recognizing the barriers that stand between you and your well-being. Spoiler: The problem is not you. **Part 2 shows you how the game is rigged and how to play by your own rules.**

Part 3: Wax On, Wax Off

In the original *The Karate Kid* movie, Mr. Miyagi teaches Danny LaRusso the art of karate by having him wax his car. "Wax on," Mr. Miyagi instructs, rotating his palm clockwise. "Wax off," he says, rotating his other palm counterclockwise. "Don't forget to breathe," he adds. Danny's training also includes sanding the deck, staining the fence, and painting the house.

Why the repetitive, mundane tasks? Because in the mundane lie the protective gestures that help us grow strong enough to defend ourselves and the people we love. **Part 3 is about what you can do every day to grow mighty and conquer burnout: Connect with the people and things you love, rest, and cultivate self-compassion.**

Appendix

There is also an appendix at the very end, where you'll find support in case you are confused by some of the phrases we use as instructions. For example, we often say "listen to your body" because it's a foundational part of this work, and it comes naturally to some people. Many of us, however, have no idea what that means. The good news is that listening to your body is a learnable skill. Anyone can do it and we'll show you how. The same goes for "mindfulness" and "brainstorming." We didn't want to take for granted that everyone just magically knows what these things are or how to do them . . . because Amelia didn't, and we figure she's not the only one.

Before We Dive In, a Word on Coping

When there's so much going on that you don't have time to work through a series of worksheets, there's coping. Our definition of "coping" is: making this moment tolerable.

Coping strategies are an important part of preventing and recovering from burnout. If we think of burnout as a wound, it's easy to understand why we need to stop the bleeding, protect the injury, and ease the pain to allow healing. Pain causes stress, and stress causes pain, so let's just cut out that self-fulfilling situation and allow ourselves to ease the pain from time to time.

Yes, the goal of this workbook is to create long-term, overall healing, but sometimes you just need the moment to be more comfortable. You probably already know what your default coping strategies are. Let's look at the balance between the good consequences and the not-so-good consequences of some coping strategies, so you can make informed decisions about what will work for you. (For an in-depth example, see "How to Eat Your Feelings" in chapter 5.)

Coping Strategies

Here's a chart with some examples of coping strategies, their potential outcomes, and space to write your own.

In the blank space, identify one thing you notice yourself doing to cope with stress. Next, think of the good things it leads to, then of the not-so-good things it could also lead to. Reflect on what this means. (10 min)

Coping Strategy	Good Outcomes	Not-So-Good Outcomes	Reflections
Drinking alcohol	Temporarily numbing. Can be a connecting activity when shared in a community. Can be done at home. Very easy, basically zero effort.	Can interfere with judgment, which can lead to relationship conflicts or dangerous behaviors like driving. Can't be done while parenting. Interferes with sleep. Damages liver. Can dangerously interact with medications and supplements. Expensive.	An occasional drink or two, especially with a friend, can loosen a tight knot of stress, but this strategy is to be used with extreme caution and explicit limitations.
Binge-watching comfort TV	Temporarily numbing. Can enable cathartic laughter or crying. Can be done with friends or family. Can be done at home. Very easy, zero effort. Inexpensive or even free.	Time-consuming. Can isolate you from friends or family. Can't be done while kids need attention.	This strategy is useful when there is time, or when it can be shared with others.

Coping Strategy	Good Outcomes	Not-So-Good Outcomes	Reflections
Going for a run	Cathartic, completes the stress response cycle. Good for the heart, digestion, and mood. Can be done with others or alone.	Time-consuming. Must be done outside the house and requires tolerable weather. Otherwise, requires expensive indoor equipment or gym membership. Can't be done while parenting, except in limited circumstances. Hard on the body (exacerbates arthritis or aggravates old injuries). High effort.	This is a good strategy, but it requires a lot of resources.

Reflect on your go-to strategies that you wrote. Is this something you'll continue doing or do you want to balance your relationship to it?

_____

_____

_____

_____

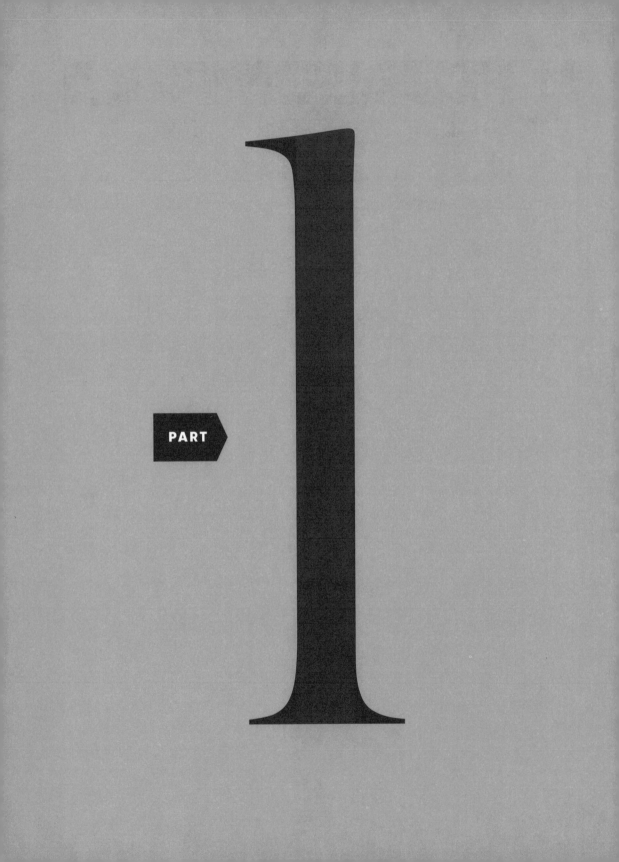

PART

1

WHAT YOU *TAKE* WITH YOU

CHAPTER 1

Complete the Cycle

Reflect Before You Read

It's helpful to notice what preconceptions you have about a topic before learning more about it.

What do you believe about stress? What is it and how do we relieve it? Have you believed differently in the past? Where have you learned about stress? How and why have your ideas changed? (5 min)

What Is Stress? Stress is the neurological and physiological shift that happens in your body when you encounter a potential threat. It's an evolutionary adaptation that activates a generic "stress response," a cascade of neurological and hormonal activities that initiate physiological changes to help you survive. This can feel like your heart racing, shortness of breath, tense muscles, and more.

Stressors are what activate the stress response in your body. They can be anything you see, hear, smell, touch, taste, or imagine could do you harm. There are external stressors: work, money, family, time, cultural norms and expectations, experiences of discrimination, and so on. And there are less tangible, internal stressors: self-criticism, body image, identity, memories, and The Future. In different ways and to different degrees, all these things may be interpreted by your body as potential threats.

Unless you can fight or flight your way out of a problem, dealing with stress is a separate process from dealing with the things that cause it. To deal with stress, you you have to complete the stress response cycle.

Your body is adapted to experience stress as a natural cycle just like all our other cycles—breathing, circulation, digestion, etc. Just like those other cycles, problems happen if the stress cycle is interrupted. That's why stress is not the enemy. Getting stuck is the enemy.

What Is the Stress Response Cycle?

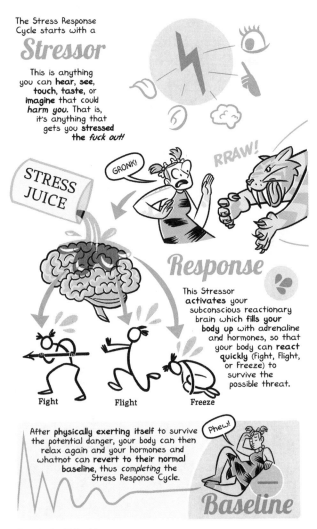

The Stress Response Cycle starts with a

Stressor

This is anything you can **hear, see, touch, taste,** or **imagine** that could **harm you.** That is, it's anything that gets you **stressed the fuck out!**

STRESS JUICE

GRONK!

RRAW!

Response

This Stressor **activates** your subconscious reactionary brain which **fills your body up** with adrenaline and hormones, so that your body can **react quickly** (Fight, Flight, or Freeze) to survive the possible threat.

Fight

Flight

Freeze

After physically **exerting itself** to survive the potential danger, your body can then relax again and your hormones and whatnot can **revert to their normal baseline,** thus *completing* the Stress Response Cycle.

Phew!

Baseline

Comic by Erika Moen

So, you respond to that pressing email, but then what? Just because you've dealt with the stressor doesn't mean you've dealt with the stress itself. The "threat" may be gone, but you haven't done anything your body recognizes as a cue that you're safe. It's stuck in the middle of a stress response cycle. Your whole body is affected—not just the cardiovascular and respiratory symptoms you may be consciously aware of. Have you experienced digestive problems when you're stressed? That's because your digestive system is affected by the stress response. Have you ever gotten sick when you're stressed? That's because your immune system takes a back seat when you're in fight-or-flight mode. Have you ever gotten a breakout when you're stressed? That's because the stress response includes hormones that alter your hair follicles and oil glands. This is how chronically activated stress response can lead to illness. So, let's fix that. But first, let's talk about why we aren't already completing the stress response cycle.

Why We Get Stuck

We get stuck because our stressors are chronic, because we're told it's "socially inappropriate" to express our emotions, because it's safer not to react, or because we've been told so many times that our feelings aren't real or valid that we've started to believe it.

And then there's "freeze." Freeze is a last-ditch response by your nervous system, when it calculates that the fight-or-flight reaction won't save you. Your nervous system stops in its tracks and shuts you down. And the freeze response is stigmatized, so survivors of trauma question themselves if they freeze. "Why didn't I fight back?" they ask themselves. "Why didn't I just run?" As if the choice to freeze was conscious. And then the stigma becomes a reason to stay stuck.

But freeze is chosen by the oldest, most survival-oriented part of your brain, way below the level of conscious awareness. It's heroic. It saves lives. And just like all the other times your stress response gets interrupted, you need to complete the cycle in a separate process before dealing with the thing that initiated the cycle.

The Feels

What comes after freezing can feel scary if you don't know what it is. Your body may shake, shudder, or otherwise respond involuntarily along with waves of rage, panic, and shame. This is what we call "the Feels."

You might try to fight it or control it, but it's nothing to fear. It's a normal, healthy part of completing the cycle. It's how adrenaline and cortisol that built up in the bloodstream get purged, the same way that running to safety purges those chemicals. It will end on its own, usually in just a few minutes.

Trust your body. The sensations may bring awareness of their origins, or they may not; either way, it doesn't matter. Awareness and insight are not required for the Feels to move through you and out of you. Crying for no discernible reason? Great! Just notice any apparently causeless emotions or sensations or trembling and say, "Ah. There's some Feels."

How stress is currently at play in your life. (15 min)

Right now, you're probably thinking of things that cause you stress. Describe a specific, recent time when you felt overwhelmed. What happened and how did your body feel?

_____

_____

_____

_____

Drawing on that experience, list the specific stressors that activated your stress response. How did you engage with them? Did you go into fight-or-flight mode? Did you freeze?

_____

_____

_____

_____

What happened after the event you described above? How did you feel? What did you do?

_____

_____

_____

_____

Have you ever experienced an instance of freezing or getting stuck? What happened? How did you feel physically and emotionally?

_____

_____

_____

_____

After a stressful event or an instance of freezing, have you experienced the Feels? Describe what that was like.

_____

_____

_____

_____

When or where or with whom do you feel free or safe to express your emotions?

_____

_____

_____

_____

How Do I Know If I've Completed the Cycle?

We get asked this all the time. It's like knowing when you're full after a meal, or like knowing when you've had an orgasm. Your body tells you and some people have an easier time recognizing it than others. You might experience it as a shift in mood or mental state or a release of physical tension—you may breathe more deeply, and your thoughts may relax. Pay attention to how you feel, and when it happens, you'll know. The good news here is that you've probably experienced it before, even if only in a low-intensity way.

Don't worry if you're not sure you can recognize when you've "completed" the cycle. Especially if you've spent a lot of years—like your whole life, maybe—holding on to your worry or anger. All you need to do is recognize that you feel incrementally better than you felt before you started.

Note: If "feeling your feelings" and "listening to your body" seem like meaningless phrases, or you just have no idea how to go about doing them, there are specific instructions in Appendix II!

How to Complete the Cycle

There are lots of ways. Not all of them will work for you, and none of them work for everyone. You probably already know some of the things that work for you, and you'll recognize them below.

Cycle-Completing Activity	Defined As	Example	Most Effective When
Moving your body	Physical activity is the single most efficient strategy for completing the stress response cycle. Any movement at all can help remind your body that it can move you from danger to safety. If it's effective for you, get your body moving enough to breathe deeply for 20 to 60 minutes a day, most days of the week.	Sweat it out by running, swimming, biking, or dancing to Beyoncé in your kitchen.	You have access to it, and you need to remind your brain that your body is a safe place to live.
Sleeping	Your brain practices and completes experiences from the past, helping you process stress (among all the other good things sleep does for us).	Probably 7 to 9 hours—in one continuous lump or in multiple chunks, during the part of the day when your body asks for it, depending on whether you're an early bird or a night owl.	You are living in a human body. If you change only one thing in your life after using this workbook, let it be getting adequate sleep.
Breathing	Deep breathing so that your belly expands and contracts.	Breathe in slowly to a count of 5, hold that breath for a count of 5, slowly exhale for a count of 10, and pause for a count of 5. Repeat 5 times.	Your stress isn't that high, or when you just need to siphon off the very worst of the stress so you can get through a difficult situation, after which you'll do something more hardcore.
Engaging in positive social interaction	Casual but friendly interactions with another person.	Have a polite conversation with your seatmate or say "Nice day" to the barista when you buy your coffee.	Your brain needs a reminder that the world is a safe place.

Cycle-Completing Activity	Defined As	Example	Most Effective When
Showing affection	Deeper connection with a loving presence who likes, respects, and trusts you, and whom you like, respect, and trust. Specifically, an action—a long kiss or hug—that tells your body that you are safe with your community.	Kiss your partner for 6 seconds. Hug someone you love and trust for 20 full seconds, while both of you are supporting your own weight. Pet a cat or play with a dog.	You are looking for an immediate shift from a state of anxiety to a state of safety.
Laughing	Loud, silly, abdomen-aching, helpless laughter.	Belly laugh with another person—or even reminisce about times you've laughed together.	You want to relieve stress in the easiest, most fun way possible.
Having a big ol' cry	Crying may not change the situation that caused your stress, but it helps you complete the cycle.	The crying may just happen on its own, or you can access it by watching your favorite tear-jerker movie.	You are looking to move from feelings of overwhelm and stuckness into a state of release and relief.
Expressing yourself creatively	Making a thing just for the pleasure of making it can move difficult feelings from inside your body out to a safe place—into a song, poem, mural, sculpture, scarf, meal, etc.	Sing, dance, write, recite, build, carve, cook, knit, paint, draw, etc.	You have the opportunity to dedicate time and resources to making things.
Engaging your imagination	Whether you imagine a thing, or it's actually happening in the world, your brain acts very similarly. This means that you can move your body through a stress cycle using your imagination alone.	Read a book, watch a movie, or play a game with the kind of heroic ending that makes you want to cheer and tell people about it! (Just staring at comfort TV is numbing rather than cycle completing.)	You get carried away by stories. Also convenient if you are limited in engaging in other cycle-completing activities (i.e., you're on a train or you have really low energy).

What do you want to do to complete the stress response cycle?

Brainstorm the stuff you like to do or want to try in the below categories. It can be anything that makes you feel good. Remember positive experiences you've had and identify specific examples. Write them in as many categories as they fit. (15 min)

Category	Possible Activities	Positive Experiences
Moving your body		
Sleeping		
Breathing		
Engaging in positive social interaction		
Showing affection		
Laughing		
Having a big ol' cry		
Expressing yourself creatively		
Engaging your imagination		

A particular combination of activities comes up again and again in people's responses: moving in time with others toward a shared goal. We call it "the Magic Trick." It's physical activity, connection with others, and connecting to something larger than yourself all in one. Go back to your chart and circle (or highlight or just recognize) anything that gives you (or could give you) that uplifted feeling that you're one with the universe. Here are some examples:

going out dancing

marching in a protest

playing a team sport

participating in worship

attending a fan convention

singing or playing an instrument (especially in an ensemble)

training for the military

attending a game or movie or concert with a crowd of other cheering fans

Can you remember a time when you did one of those things and it seemed to lift you up and leave you feeling amazing? Write about it below.

Now that you've thought through the activities that complete the stress response cycle for you, use this space to fill in words or pictures that express how you've felt when you've done some cycle-completing activities. How do you know you've completed the cycle?

Barriers

We've established what you can do to complete the stress response cycle. But if you're here doing these exercises, there are probably reasons you're not doing those things already. We want to recognize that those barriers are real, it's not your fault that you haven't already overcome them, and you're not alone.

Everyone we know is swamped by personal, mental, physical, logistical, and social barriers that come between them and their own well-being. Still, everyone can also find a way through those barriers to access the resources they need.

Every chapter after this one has more ideas and strategies for overcoming the barriers that stand between you and your own well-being.

TO WRAP UP THE CHAPTER: Think of some stories, songs, art works, processes, etc. that support or reinforce the ideas in this chapter. (10 min)

OUR EXAMPLE:

Warrior Poet: A Biography of Audre Lorde by Alexis De Veaux (book)

YOUR EXAMPLES:

Wellness happens when your body is a place of safety for you, even when your body is not necessarily in a safe place. You can be well, even during the times when you don't feel good.

CHAPTER 2

#Persist

Reflect Before You Read

It's helpful to notice what preconceptions you have about a topic before learning more about it.

Does frustration seem like a good thing or a bad thing? Productive or disruptive? What is frustration exactly, and what causes it? What can you do about it? (5 min)

What Causes Stress?

Chapter 1 was about the stress in your body. This chapter is about managing the things that cause that stress. It's about knowing—when you're past the edge of your capabilities—how to persist and when to quit. Specifically, it's about what we call "the Monitor," the brain mechanism that manages the gap between where we are and where we are going. (Technically, it's called the "discrepancy-reducing/-increasing feedback loop" and "criterion velocity," but people fall asleep immediately when we say that, so we just call it "the Monitor.") Exactly what this looks like is different for everyone, but it impacts every domain of life, from parenthood to career success to friendships to body image. And for women, the gap quickly becomes a chasm.

In this chapter, we'll explain how the Monitor works, and why it sometimes breaks down. Then we'll practice evidence-based strategies for every frustration and every failure, from traffic jams to tenure.

The Monitor knows

1. what your goal is.

2. how much effort you're investing in that goal.

3. how much progress you're making.

It keeps a running tally of your effort-to-progress ratio, and it has a strong opinion about what that ratio should be. There are so many ways a plan can go wrong, some of which you can control and some of which you can't, and all of which will frustrate your Monitor.

For example, imagine you're working toward a simple goal: driving to the mall. You know it usually takes about, say, twenty minutes. If you're getting all green lights and you're zipping right along, that feels nice, right? You're making progress more quickly and easily than your Monitor expects, and that feels great. **Less effort, more progress equals a satisfied Monitor.**

But suppose you get stuck at a traffic light because another driver wasn't paying attention. You feel a little annoyed and frustrated, and maybe you try to get around that jerk before the next light. But once you've hit one red light, you end up stuck at every traffic light, and with each stop, your frustration burns a little hotter. It's already been twenty minutes, and you're only halfway to the mall. "Annoyed and frustrated" escalates to "pissed off." Then you get on the highway, and there's an accident! While ambulances and police come and go, you sit there, parked on the highway for forty minutes, fuming and boiling and swearing never to go to the mall again. **High effort, little progress equals an enraged Monitor.**

If you sit there long enough, an enormous emotional shift happens inside you. Your Monitor switches its assessment of your goal from "attainable" to "unattainable," and pushes you off an emotional cliff, into a *pit of despair*. Lost in helplessness, your brain abandons hope, and you sit in your car sobbing, because all you want to do now is go home, and there's nothing you can do but sit there and wait.

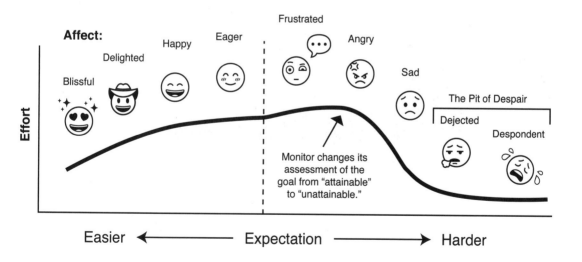

What Kind of Stressor?

There are two flavors of stressors: the ones you can control and the ones you can't.

The stressors you can control include busy schedules, managing medication, relationship challenges, etc. These are all difficult to live with, but you can take concrete steps to manage them and even eliminate them.

The stressors you can't control may go away on their own, or they may be things you'll need to manage for the foreseeable future. For example, we live in an unfair economic system that protects the wealth of the rich and allows them to exploit the poor, making the gap between the two groups grow wider than ever. That's a stressor that affects your life in a lot of different ways, and it's almost certainly not going away in your lifetime. There are concrete actions you can take to try to create long-term change but that change will be slow. The arc of history may bend toward justice, but it doesn't bend quickly. So, we also need to learn strategies for managing their immediate impacts on our lives, which we'll talk about next.

Sort Your Stressors (5 min)

For now, let's check in with the things that cause you stress, and notice which ones you have some immediate control over, and which ones you don't, starting with a few examples.

Fill in your stressors below and get as specific or as broad as you like.

Stressors You Can Control	Stressors You Can't Control
Cooking dinner every night	Patriarchy
Your overflowing bathroom cabinet	Your boss's condescending attitude
The fly in the room	The traffic jam on the way to work

You might be feeling a little stressed after this exercise, so take a moment to turn toward the stress in your body and let it complete its cycle.

As you were writing out the list of stressors you can control, you were probably also thinking of the many things you would have to do to manage them or wondering if there are YouTube videos about how to fix them. That's the good news about stressors you can control—you can take concrete steps, and there are many resources widely available to help!

Planful Problem-Solving

If you write to-do lists, keep calendars, or follow a budget, you know what planful problem-solving entails: You analyze the problem, make a plan based on your analysis, and then execute the plan.

(The least intuitive part of planful problem-solving is managing the stress caused by the problems and the solving. As we learned in chapter 1, what works to manage your stressor will rarely help you manage the stress, so remember to build completing the cycle into your plan.)

Practicing Planning (15 min)

Choose some of the items from your list of stressors you can control on the previous page and write out your plans for dealing with them. It's not cheating to use a stressor and a plan you've already accomplished, but take a few minutes to recognize how many steps it took, and how many resources you needed. And remember to include cycle completing in your plan.

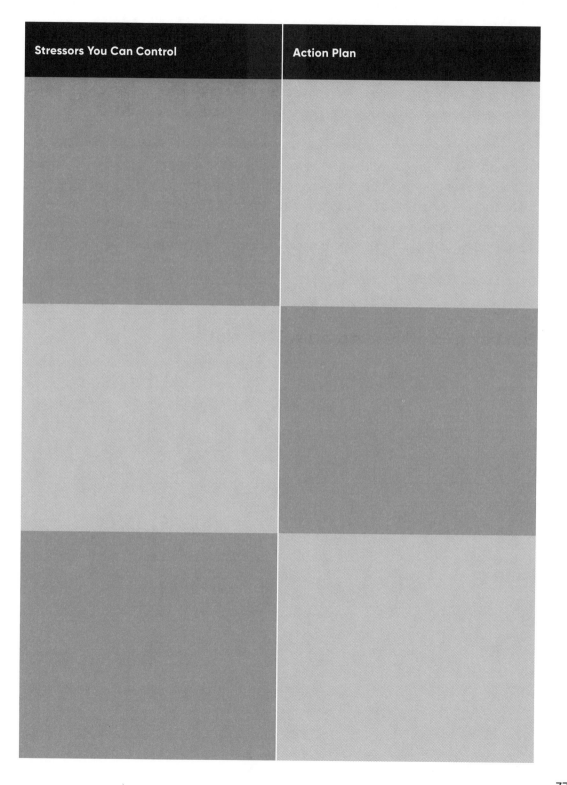

Stressors You Can Control	Action Plan

Dealing with Stressors You Can't Control

They say you can solve any problem or eliminate any obstacle if you "want it enough" or "believe!" If those strategies work for you, great! For the rest of us, here are evidence-based solutions for managing the stressors beyond your control.

The tool here is "positive reappraisal." Positive reappraisal involves recognizing that the challenge you're facing is worth it. It means acknowledging that the effort, discomfort, frustration, unanticipated obstacles, and even repeated failures have value—not just because they are steps toward a worthwhile goal, but because you reframe difficulties as opportunities for growth and learning. Just identifying the worthiness of your difficulty is enough to change the monitor's ratio of effort to progress.

It's that easy! And, that difficult.

Practicing Positive Reappraisal (10 min)

What are some of your biggest challenges with uncontrollable stressors right now?

How are these challenges also opportunities for growth and learning?

_____

_____

_____

_____

_____

_____

_____

_____

When you think you need more "grit," what you really need is help. And when you think you need persistence, what you really need is kindness.

Compare the value of the opportunities for growth and learning to the amount of challenges of the uncontrollable stressors. Does dealing with those stressors feel worth it?

_____

_____

_____

_____

_____

_____

_____

_____

_____

Redefine Winning

Planful problem-solving and positive reappraisal are evidence-based ways to change the effort you invest as you move toward a goal. They'll reduce your frustration by keeping you motivated and moving forward. However, suppose you do all that, and it works, but your progress is not meeting your Monitor's expectations about how difficult it will be or how long it will take?

When you're frustrated by the slow or interrupted progress toward achieving your goal, and planful problem-solving and positive reappraisal don't help with the frustration, you need to redefine what it means to "win" at this goal.

Find Your New Wins (15 min)

What is a goal or project you are struggling with or thinking about a lot?

_____

_____

_____

_____

_____

What is it about this goal that frustrates your Monitor? Does it seem unattainable? Do you feel ambivalent about it? Was it someone else's dopey idea? Does part of this goal make you feel helpless? Are there too many frustrating, yet unavoidable, obstacles between you and "winning"?

_____

_____

_____

_____

_____

Brainstorm at least twenty options for definitions of "winning" that will satisfy your Monitor. Make sure you have plenty of silly, impractical ideas, as well as a few that could work. For example, when it comes to parenting, maybe "winning" looks like your child graduating from high school or learning to tie their shoes. (If you like, try setting a timer for 10 minutes and challenge yourself to keep writing ideas the whole time, no matter how bad those ideas seem.)

NOTE: Brainstorming works best when you don't filter! For some people, it also works better when you collaborate; if that's you, ask a friend to help. For more suggestions about effective brainstorming, see Appendix III.

1. _____
2. _____
3. _____
4. _____
5. _____
6. _____
7. _____
8. _____
9. _____
10. _____
11. _____
12. _____
13. _____
14. _____
15. _____
16. _____
17. _____
18. _____
19. _____
20. _____

Now choose your three favorite wins from the list you brainstormed on page 41 and score them based on how well they please your Monitor. As an example, we've redefined the goal "Smash the patriarchy" into the new win of "Buy from women-owned businesses."

Specific Goal	SOON	CERTAIN	SPECIFIC
	When will you know you've succeeded? (Your goal should be achievable without requiring patience.)	How confident are you that you can succeed? (Your goal should be within your control.)	As opposed to general. (You should be able to visualize precisely what success will look like.)
Example Win: Buy from women-owned businesses	I can do it as soon as I have an opportunity to buy a product or service.	I can 100 percent do this by searching the internet for women-owned businesses.	Women-owned, not men-owned. Buy, not just browse.
Win #1:			
Win #2:			
Win #3:			

CONCRETE	POSITIVE	PERSONAL
Measurable. How will you know you've succeeded? (There is an external indication that you have succeeded.)	What improvement will you experience when you win? (Your goal should be something that feels good, not just something that avoids suffering.)	Does this goal matter to you? How much does it matter? (Tailor your goal so that it matters to you.)
If I acquire a thing I needed, and I acquired it from a business owned by women!	I'll use my resources to lift up other women.	It matters because business is one of the places where women face more barriers than men, and I have the power to support change.

When to Give Up

The Monitor has a pivot point, when it switches its assessment of your goal from "attainable" to "unattainable." You may find yourself oscillating between pushing onward and giving up, between frustrated rage—"This goal is attainable and screw these jerks who are getting in my way!"—and helpless despair—"I can't do it, I give up, everything is terrible!"

If you want to understand when you should give up, all you have to do is write four lists:

1. What are the benefits of continuing?

2. What are the benefits of stopping?

3. What are the costs of continuing?

4. What are the costs of stopping?

Practicing Quitting (20 min)

Think of something you're considering whether to continue or quit. Fill out the Decision Grid on the opposite page. Then look at those four lists and decide based on your estimates of maximizing benefit and minimizing cost. Remember to consider both the immediate and longer-term costs and benefits. And if you decide to continue, remember to include completing the cycle in your plan.

DECISION GRID

Should I continue or quit: _____

(e.g., my job, my relationship, my diet, my place of worship, my substance use . . .)

Continuing	Quitting

Benefits / Immediate

Benefits / Immediate

Benefits / Longer-term

Benefits / Longer-term

Costs / Immediate

Costs / Immediate

Costs / Longer-term

Costs / Longer-term

There are endless
examples of people
not achieving their
specific goal but achieving
something important,
something world-
changing, along their
path to failure.

This is the last time in the workbook we'll focus on dealing with stressors; and there's a reason we spend so little time on them. We're here to help you with the most effective tools in the widest variety of circumstances, starting with the resources you carry with you as part of your humanity, and concluding with the connections that support you. When you know how to use those internal resources, you'll have more energy and comfort to address the things that cause stress not only in your life, but also in the lives of those around you.

TO WRAP UP THE CHAPTER: Think of some stories, songs, art works, processes, etc. that support or reinforce the ideas in this chapter. (10 min)

OUR EXAMPLE:
Up (movie)

YOUR EXAMPLES:

CHAPTER 3

Meaning

Reflect Before You Read

It's helpful to notice what preconceptions you have about a topic before learning more about it.

What do you believe about "meaning in life"? Where and from whom did you learn what meaning is? How has your understanding of meaning changed during your life? Where does meaning come from? (5 min)

Every Disney heroine has an "I Want" song, in which she explains what is missing in her life. Moana feels called by the ocean. Tiana is "almost there," saving money to start her own restaurant. Belle wants "adventure in the great wide somewhere." The tradition goes all the way back to Snow White singing "Someday My Prince Will Come." You can chart the progress of women in America by the things Disney heroines sing about in their "I Want" songs. Although what they sing about changes, there is one constant: A heroine feels called by something.

Now, just as most of us don't spontaneously burst into song (though some of us do!), most of us don't lead lives of epic heroism and high-stakes adventure. We have jobs and school. We have kids to feed, a bathtub to scrub, an inbox to clear, not to mention novels to read and shows to catch up on. But like all heroines, we thrive when we are answering the call of something larger than ourselves. This chapter is about meaning as a power you carry inside that helps you resist and recover from burnout.

What Is Meaning? "Meaning," in short, is the nourishing experience of feeling like we're connected to something larger than ourselves. It helps us thrive when things are going well, and it helps us cope when things go wrong in our lives. So, where does meaning come from?

You Make Meaning

You may be used to hearing about meaning as something we "search for" or "discover," and sometimes people experience it that way—as a sudden revelation that descends upon them from on high, or a treasure that they find after years of following the map. But rarely is meaning something that we find at the end of a long, hard journey. For most of us, meaning is what sustains us on that journey, no matter what we find at the end. Meaning is not found; it is made. To make meaning, the research tells us, engage with something larger than yourself. This "Something Larger"—like a god you believe in or a dream you have for the future—is your source of meaning.

A woman's need for "meaning in life" is not fundamentally different from a man's, but the obstacles that stand between women and their sense of meaning *are* different.

Find Your Something Larger

Some people know exactly what their Something Larger is, and others take years to figure it out. There is no predictable way for everyone to find it for themselves. The common thread is an inner voice that you can hear if you stop and listen. Everyone has it. Hear that? The steady rhythm in the center of your chest? Some folks have an easier time recognizing it than others. Here are a few options for identifying your Something Larger. (We can't give you a time guideline for this one. Some folks will already have this answer at their fingertips, others might need a few days. Most are probably in between.)

Look at photos of yourself from when you've felt your happiest and best. Write about what you notice. What are you doing? Who are you with? How might you harness that energy now?

_____

_____

_____

_____

_____

Think of a time when you experienced an intense sense of meaning or purpose or "alignment" or whatever it feels like for you. What were you doing? What was it about that activity that created this sense of meaning?

_____

_____

_____

_____

_____

_____

What makes you feel most powerful? Is there something you enjoy doing that feels most like what you're meant to do?

_____

_____

_____

_____

_____

_____

Try writing your own obituary or a "life summary" through the eyes of a grandchild or a student.

Ask your closest friends to describe the "real you," the characteristics of your personality and your life that are at the core of your best self. Make a list of the words they use below. If it feels too weird to ask others, try writing these yourself.

1. _____
2. _____
3. _____
4. _____
5. _____
6. _____

Imagine that someone you care about is going through a dark moment in their life—they've experienced significant loss and feel helpless and isolated (the two things that drain us of meaning fastest). As your best self, write that person a letter to support them through this difficult time.

Dear_____,

_____

_____

_____

_____

_____

_____

_____

_____

_____

_____

_____

_____

_____

_____

_____

Love,_____

Now reread this letter. It's for you.

You Make Meaning

Research has found that meaning is most likely to come from three kinds of sources:

1. Pursuit and achievement of ambitious goals that leave a legacy (e.g., finding a cure for HIV or making the world a better place for kids).

2. Service to the divine or other spiritual calling (e.g., attaining spiritual liberation and union with Akal or glorifying God with thoughts, words, and deeds).

3. Loving, emotionally intimate connection with others (e.g., raising kids so they know they're loved no matter what or loving and supporting a partner with authenticity and kindness).

Many sources of meaning are a combination of all three, and if your Something Larger falls outside these three categories, that's cool, too. In terms of your personal well-being, there is no right or wrong source of meaning; there's just whatever gives you the feeling that your life has a positive impact.

How Do *You* Make Meaning? (10 min)

On the opposite page, identify goals, acts of service, and ways of connecting with others currently at work in your own life. Include ideas for new possibilities. Feel free to pull from your answers in the previous exercises.

Legacy	Service	Connection

When Terrible Things Happen

Sometimes, terrible things happen, leaving us feeling trapped and convinced that nothing we do will make a difference. How can people continue to engage with their Something Larger in the face of terrible things—even in the face of terrible things that separate them from their Something Larger? The key is: **You can never be separated from your Something Larger, because it is inside you.**

In such times of crisis, we must turn inward and confront difficult feelings with kindness and compassion.

Write Your Origin Story (40 min)

Meaning is not made by the terrible thing you experienced; it is made by the ways you survive. This process might hurt. That's actually another part of what makes it effective: It allows your body to practice feeling the feelings of past wounds, to learn that those feelings are not dangerous, and to complete the incomplete stress response cycles activated all those years ago. It starts with your willingness to look, to risk the discomfort of paying attention to what you thought was only negative, and to learn to see it with nonjudgment, curiosity, and even compassion.

Rewrite the narrative of your experience, focusing on the lessons and strengths you gained through adversity. Write your story, answering these questions:

1. **What parts of the adversity were uncontrollable by you?** (For example, other people and their choices, cultural norms, your life circumstances at the time, your age and prior experience, the weather.)

2. **What did you do in the moment to survive the adversity?** (Hint: We know for sure that you did successfully survive the adversity, because here you are. Yay!)

3. **After the adversity passed, what resources did you leverage to continue to survive?** (Be specific: This may include practical resources like money or information; social resources like friends; your ability to seek, find, and accept help; or emotional resources like persistence, self-soothing, and optimism.)

NOTE: For most people, the most effective version of this exercise will take about half an hour, but if it helps you, spend a few days on it. (For folks dealing with trauma, this might be an exercise to accomplish with a friend or therapist.)

Once you have your story, take a moment to write about a time when those resources empowered you to overcome a subsequent difficulty.

Now write a summary and any other thoughts you might have.

Even though I couldn't control _____ ,
(ADVERSITY)

I managed to _____ **, and then I used**
(SURVIVAL TACTIC)

_____ **to grow stronger.**
(RESOURCE)

After that, I could _____ .
(SKILL/WIN/INSIGHT)

Other thoughts:

_____

_____

_____

_____

_____

_____

_____

_____

_____

_____

_____

_____

_____

_____

_____

_____

_____

_____

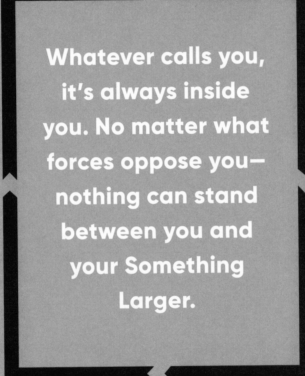

Whatever calls you, it's always inside you. No matter what forces oppose you— nothing can stand between you and your Something Larger.

Maybe everyone around you disagrees. Maybe your family wants you to stay home—or leave home. Maybe even your mentors are skeptical, and only your grandmother who is also a mystical stingray agrees with you. Still, you hear it over the noise of implicit cultural expectations, and through the suffering of violence and injustice. You know; you hear the call in your heart.

Write an encouraging note, reminder, or promise to yourself to be true to your Something Larger, no matter what anyone else thinks. Include how you will make space to connect with that calling regularly. Tear it out and carry it with you or hang it somewhere you'll be able to see every day.

TO WRAP UP THE CHAPTER: Think of some stories, songs, art works, processes, etc. that support or reinforce the ideas in this chapter. (10 min)

OUR EXAMPLES:

Moana (movie)
Unravel (video game)

YOUR EXAMPLES:

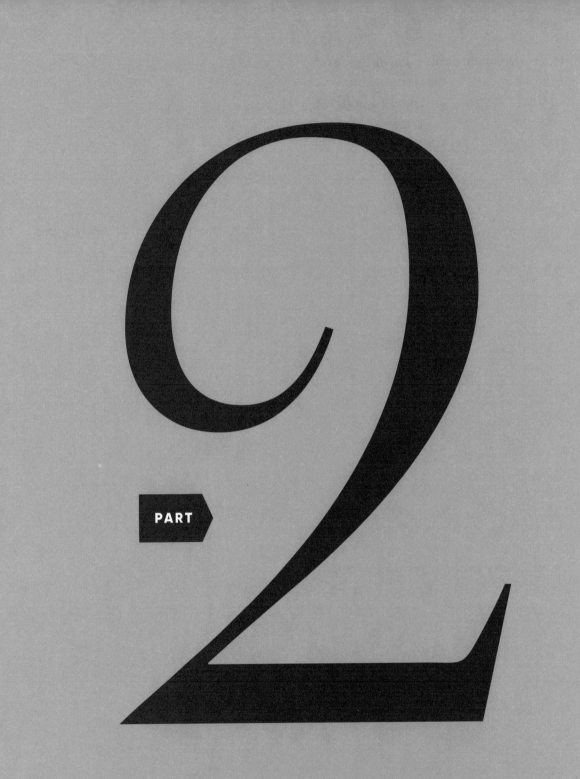

PART

THE
REAL
ENEMY

CHAPTER 4

The Game Is Rigged

Reflect Before You Read

It's helpful to notice what preconceptions you have about a topic before learning more about it.

What does the word "patriarchy" mean to you? Where did you first learn about it, and from whom? How do you feel about it and why do you feel that way? (5 min)

The Patriarchy (Ugh)

We know. The word "patriarchy" (ugh) makes many people uncomfortable. If you're one of those people, that's completely fine. You don't need to accept the word, or use it, to recognize the symptoms of living in it.

Women and girls—especially women and girls of color—are systematically excluded from government and other systems of power. The game is rigged. It's called "patriarchy" (ugh) and it says it doesn't exist. It says that if we struggle, it's our own fault for not being "good enough." Which is gaslighting.

One of the things that makes this easy to overlook is Human Giver Syndrome—the contagious belief that women have a moral obligation to give everything, every moment of their lives, every drop of their energy, to the care of others, no matter the cost to themselves—which thrives in the patriarchy, the way mold thrives in damp basements.

Giving and being a giver are not dangerous or harmful when you're surrounded by other givers. That's actually a perfect way to create an equitable society where no one falls through the cracks, because everyone feels an obligation to care for others around them—if you start to burn out, someone will turn to you and offer care. Human Giver Syndrome becomes a danger in the context of a system that maintains political and social hierarchy that only gives power to people who conform to a narrow, arbitrary, socially constructed ideal—namely rich, white, thin, straight, able-bodied, college-educated, neurotypical, cis men, etc.

You might have Human Giver Syndrome if you believe:

1. You have a moral obligation, at all times, to be pretty, happy, calm, generous, and attentive to the needs of others.

2. If you fail in your moral obligation to be pretty, happy, calm, generous, and attentive to the needs of others, at all times, then you are a failure.

3. Being a failure means you deserve punishment. And if no one is around to punish you, then you'll do it yourself.

4. These are normal and true ideas.

Notice the Giving in Your Life (15 min)

How does the idea of Human Giver Syndrome resonate with you? What are the ways it shows up in your own life, relationships, or career?

_____

_____

_____

_____

_____

_____

_____

_____

_____

Who are the givers in your life who care for your well-being as much as you care for theirs? Who are the people in your life who seem to feel entitled to your time, life, and body? Describe the differences between your relationships with them. What would it be like to focus on your relationships with the givers, and reduce your investment in relationships with the rest?

_____

_____

_____

_____

_____

_____

_____

Go for a walk. Scream into a pillow. Or, as Carrie Fisher put it, "Take your broken heart, make it into art." Reverse the effects of helplessness by creating a context where you can do a thing.

Complete the Cycle: Feeling About the Patriarchy

As Gloria Steinem wrote, "The truth will set you free, but first it will piss you off!" Seeing the rigged game isn't a neutral experience; you'll probably feel some feelings about it as you go through the world spotting the ways the game is rigged and the ways the world is lying to you about the ways the game is rigged. These feelings are uncomfortable, and when they get really intense, it's tempting to ignore them and just stop playing the game. In other words: burnout. So, let's not ignore them.

A lot of us are carrying around decades of incomplete stress response cycles because Human Giver Syndrome told us we had to be happy and calm and not make other people uncomfortable with our feelings. Remember that those feelings are cycles that happen in your body, and you need to give them that opportunity. Chapter 1 is always available as a reminder of all the things you can do to complete the stress response cycle.

Unlearning Helplessness: Do a Thing

"Learned Helpnessness" describes what happens to your nervous system when it experiences frustration and failure so many times that the monitor gives up and decides it can't attain any goals. After experiments into learned helplessness, meant to frustrate participants until their Monitors dumped them into a pit of despair, just telling a helpless human that the experiment is rigged was enough to lift them out of the pit and make them feel immediately better. But when learned helplessness has been induced during a lifetime of experience, you need to teach your nervous system that it's not helpless. How? You do something—and "something" is anything that isn't nothing. For example, lots of folks feel intense pleasure from tidying a single drawer—the rest of the desk/room/house might be swimming in mess, but that doesn't diminish the pleasure you feel the moment you look into that drawer and admire how tidy it is.

This kind of small, successful task reminds your nervous system that it isn't helpless, that it has agency and efficacy. In other words, this is about dealing with the stress in your body in a separate process from dealing with the thing that caused your stress.

Practice Unlearning Helplessness (10 min)

Think about some times in the past when things out of your individual control left you feeling overwhelmed, helpless, or like you wanted to quit (e.g., systemic racism, climate change, managing disability or chronic illness, working in an exploitative environment). What were the stressors? And what did helplessness feel like in your heart, mind, and/or body?

_____

_____

_____

_____

_____

_____

_____

_____

Recall some chores or other small-scale tasks that made you feel successful, satisfied, or proud (e.g., tidying, gardening, learning a skill, chopping firewood). What were the tasks? And what did the achievements feel like in your heart, mind, and/or body?

_____

_____

_____

_____

_____

_____

That's the feeling of unlearning helplessness! Over time, tackling small tasks can help you become ready to take on some of the larger tasks involved in making changes to those uncontrollable stressors.

When you're ready, look back at your list of stressors, and identify actions you can take to create change in your small patch of the world. If you get stuck thinking about the enormity of those problems, you can just search the internet for "what can I do about . . ." or "how do I manage . . ." and there will likely be blogs and videos and book recommendations galore. Keep a list of actions you can take to help contribute to positive change in your small patch of the world.

_____

_____

_____

_____

_____

_____

Smash

You're completing the cycle. You're *doing* things, using your body to remind yourself that you are not helpless.

Next step: Smash the patriarchy. Smash it to pieces.

You smash it by making meaning—engaging with your Something Larger in ways that heal Human Giver Syndrome.

Smashin'-Some-Patriarchy Worksheet (5 min)

My Something Larger is: _____

_____

_____

_____

Something I do to engage with my Something Larger that also smashes some patriarchy is: _____

_____

_____

_____

I'll know I smashed some patriarchy when . . . (soon, certain, specific, concrete, positive, and personal): _____

_____

_____

_____

A Word on Compassion Fatigue

The patriarchy (ugh) not only affects us directly, but it also causes harm to us indirectly as we care for others. When we experience stress on behalf of others, we may dismiss it as inconsequential or "irrational" and ignore it. Givers may spend years attending to the needs of others, while dismissing their own stress that was generated in response to witnessing those needs. The result is uncountable incomplete stress response cycles accumulating in our bodies. This accumulation leads to "compassion fatigue," and it's a primary cause of burnout among givers, including those who work in helping professions (many of which are dominated by women—teaching, social work, health care, etc.).

Signs of compassion fatigue include:

1. checking out, emotionally
   faking empathy when you know you're supposed to feel it, because you can't feel the real thing anymore

2. minimizing or dismissing suffering that isn't the most extreme
   "It's not slavery/genocide/nuclear war, so quit complaining"

3. feeling helpless, hopeless, or powerless, while also feeling personally responsible for doing more

4. staying in a bad situation, whether a workplace or a relationship, out of a sense of grandiosity
   "If I don't do it, no one will."

Noticing Your Compassion Fatigue (10 min)

What is your experience with compassion fatigue? What suffering have you witnessed while having to remain calm and helpful? What did that feel like? Did it change or add up over time?

_____

_____

_____

_____

Just reflecting on these experiences can initiate a stress response in your body. You've been practicing noticing what difficult experiences feel like in your body, and as you get better at it, you might start to notice more stress and think, "This workbook is just stressing me out more!" Don't give up. Uncomfortable feelings aren't dangerous. They're just cycles that happen in your body. Notice the discomfort, observe it, let it complete its cycle. Determine if this opportunity for learning and growth is worth it (positive reappraisal, chapter 2 FTW!).

By the way, yes, it's worth it. And it gets easier as you go, because you're getting better at it.

TO WRAP UP THE CHAPTER: Think of some stories, songs, art works, processes, etc. that support or reinforce the ideas in this chapter. (10 min)

OUR EXAMPLES:
9 to 5 (movie)
Kindred by Octavia E. Butler (book)
The Color Purple by Alice Walker (book)
The Woman Warrior: Memoirs of a Girlhood Among Ghosts
    by Maxine Hong Kingston (book)

YOUR EXAMPLES:

_____

_____

_____

_____

_____

_____

_____

_____

_____

_____

_____

_____

When you engage with
your Something Larger
and thus make meaning
in your life, you're
actually healing
Human Giver Syndrome,
both in yourself and in
the people around you.

CHAPTER 5

The Bikini Industrial Complex

Reflect Before You Read

It's helpful to notice what preconceptions you have about a topic before learning more about it.

What does the phrase "body positivity" mean to you? How do you feel when someone encourages you to "love your body?" How do you feel about your body, and when did you start feeling that way? Did you ever feel differently? Where did you learn how to feel about your body? (5 min)

_____

_____

_____

_____

_____

_____

Imagine if you didn't have to worry about conforming to the narrow, arbitrary, socially constructed ideal of what's beautiful. What if you knew that you'd be safe and loved and have unlimited access to every resource you need without having to change anything about yourself? What would that be like? (5 min)

_____

_____

_____

_____

_____

_____

_____

The Bikini Industrial Complex

The "Bikini Industrial Complex" is a hundred-billion-dollar industry that tries to convince us that our bodies are the enemy, when, in reality, the Bikini Industrial Complex itself is the enemy.

You already know that everything in the media is there to sell you thinness—the shellacked abs in advertisements for exercise equipment, the One Weird Trick to Lose Belly Fat clickbait when all you wanted was a weather forecast, and princesses played by "flawlessly" thin women in movies. It's even in our doctors' offices, decorated with the BMI chart—a piece of propaganda designed by people who profit off the weight-loss industry, codified as medical standard not by scientists but by lobbyists. The Bikini Industrial Complex has successfully created a culture of immense pressure to conform to an ideal that is literally unobtainable by almost everyone and yet is framed not just as the most beautiful, but the healthiest and most virtuous.

Remember, humans are like a herd species—and when there's danger, where's the safest place in the herd? The middle. So, if you're on the fringes of social belonging, your body can interpret this as a threat. Pressure to conform and your need to belong are not coming from your insecurity or vanity; they're coming from evolution. So, we try to fit the socially constructed ideal. This is reinforced by society itself, where there are harsh negative consequences to those who don't conform, which show up as bigotry, including racism, misogyny, ableism, and fatphobia.

Besides the negative consequences of the stress created by the pressure to conform, as well as the side effects of the things we do to try to conform (including disordered relationships with food and exercise, overspending on clothes, beauty supplies, and treatments), there is also "self-regulatory fatigue." We're using up decision-making and attention-focusing cognitive resources on choices about food, clothes, exercise, makeup, body hair, "toxins," and fretting about our bodies' failures.

Really Good News

On the day a girl is born, she may be lucky enough to have people around her who instantly welcome every roll on her body, every wrinkle on her fingers, every blotch on her skin, and each and every hair, no matter where it is on her brand-new little body. Her little body is full of needs—food, sleep, diaper changes, being held. Most of us are met, at our birth, with an enveloping, protective love that holds and cherishes every inch of our bodies. In that moment and in that love, we are flawless. Beautiful.

Picture that girl on the day of her birth, perfect and helpless and full of life, maybe held against the skin of a loving parent.

She's beautiful, right? She's perfect.

And she's you.

Here is the secret Human Giver Syndrome doesn't want you to know: Nothing has changed. No matter what has happened to that body of yours between the day you were born, beautiful and perfect, and the day you read this, your body is still beautiful and perfect. And it is still full of needs. In *Burnout*, we spend a large chunk of chapter 5 discussing the actual science behind body weight, because that's a nearly universal feature of women's stress. By the age of six, about half of girls are worried about being "too fat." By adolescence, almost all girls will have engaged in some kind of "weight control" behavior. Almost half (44 percent) of girls engaged in *unhealthy* weight-control behaviors. But, though weight-related bias called "scientific weightism" pollutes research and medical care, none of the popular ideas about body size and shape are supported by the science.

Only a very small fraction of the population can lose weight and sustain that weight loss through diet and exercise. You have a "defended weight" (heavily influenced by genetics) that your body will try to maintain no matter how you feed it and exercise it. That defended weight usually goes up with age. Also, there is very little correlation between weight and health. **You're just as likely to experience disease whether you are fat or thin.**

This is the good news: All those good things you imagined in the previous exercise can be real right now.

Reflect on your feelings about these facts. (10 min)

Do you have doubts? Do you feel frustrated? Does a part of you want to hold on to the belief that the BMI chart is a trustworthy guide to what weight is appropriate for you? Are you thinking about where you learned that you can and should lose weight, and are you wondering how so many people could possibly have been so wrong?

Is there a part of you that wants this to be true, that's glad to be freed from expectations that have burdened you for years, that hopes for a life without the worry you currently carry? Is some part of you celebrating? What is that like?

Find Your New "Weight Loss" Goal (40 min)

Back in chapter 2, we talked about "when to quit." We suggested you fill out another grid—with the immediate and longer-term benefits of keeping a goal, and immediate and longer-term benefits of letting go of a goal.

First, try the Decision Grid with whatever your current body goal is. Or you can listen to your inner voice, which has probably been begging for mercy for years. Include thoughts, feelings, and words you would use about your body in each part of the grid, as well as the reactions of other people.

Then, on the next two pages, replace it with a goal that can improve your well-being, and make you feel healthier and more confident. We call this goal "mess acceptance." You achieve it by noticing when you have contradictory thoughts and feelings about body shape and size. Those contradictions make up the mess. Your body may feel amazing and be able to accomplish amazing things; and at the same time, you may be dissatisfied with it, or recognize how it gets negatively judged by others.

Our vision of mess acceptance comes straight out of Amelia's tai chi practice. In that work, the yin-yang symbol represents the whole universe, a single entity made up of opposites that interplay, of contradictions that coexist.

DECISION GRID

Should I stay or quit: _____

_____

(e.g., my job, my relationship, my diet, my place of worship, my substance use . . .)

Staying the same	Quitting

Benefits / Immediate

Benefits / Longer-term

Benefits / Immediate

Benefits / Longer-term

Costs / Immediate

Costs / Longer-term

Costs / Immediate

Costs / Longer-term

Practice Mess Acceptance by seeing your many, sometimes contradictory feelings about your body as part of a single whole. Write out all the positive and negative thoughts and feelings you have about your body right now, and group them into the lighter or darker side of the yin-yang symbol—you choose which group goes in which side.

Then spend some time looking at the whole, recognizing that the positive and the negative coexist. Reimagining the coexistence of opposites into a single whole can rewire your brain over time, increasing your tolerance. It creates a new goal, not for you to try to conform to one side or another, but to perceive your place in the world, which is a contradictory mess of frustration, failure, and despair, as well as progress, success, and joy. (10 min, multiple times!)

To engage more of your senses in the process of mess acceptance, you can use a tai-chi gesture called "embrace tiger, return to mountain." Several practices use the same name for different gestures, but the one Amelia learned is easy, and you can do it right now:

1. Find a comfortable, stable position. We'll call this "mountain."

2. Reach toward the mess of positive and negative thoughts and feelings you listed on page 82 and scoop it up toward your face. Breathe. Observe the mess without judgment. Think to yourself, "Yep, there's the mess," and other nonjudgmental thoughts, or just notice the feelings that come up in response to the mess. The mess is "tiger."

3. Let go of your scoop of mess, then go back to your comfortable "mountain."

4. Repeat this process for as long as you can stay focused.

"Hi, Body, What Do You Need?"

Many of us have grown to be world-class ignorers of our own needs, just as we were taught to be. We don't even notice that we're ignoring our needs. Our bodies are sending us all kinds of signals, but we live from the neck up, only attending to the noise in our heads and shutting out the noise coming from the other 95 percent of our internal experiences.

Turn your attention away from the mirror and other people's bodies and notice what it feels like inside your own. Greet your internal sensations with the same kindness and compassion you practiced when you thought about the shape and size of your body.

Imagine that your body is the body of someone who needs your care, like an infant. Take a slow breath, focus on the sensation of your weight on the floor or the chair and kindly ask yourself—either out loud or quietly—the following questions. Write what comes to you in the space that follows. This exercise feels weird and wrong to a lot of us at first but give it a try. Instead of just looking at your body to evaluate her well-being (we know that you can't tell anything about a person's health by the shape or size of their body), turn to her and ask her how she feels. She can definitely tell you if you listen.

Listen to Your Body (15 min)

You may receive the answer as an instantaneous knowing, or as a physical sensation you need to interpret, or as words in your mind. But she will give you an answer.

How are you feeling?

_____

_____

_____

What do you need?

_____

_____

_____

Is anything wrong?

_____

_____

_____

_____

Are you hungry? Thirsty? What kind of food do you need?

_____

_____

_____

_____

Are you tired? How much sleep do you need, and when?

_____

_____

_____

_____

Are you lonely? Do you need loving attention, and if so, from whom? Do you need time alone?

_____

_____

_____

_____

Did any of your answers surprise you? Have you been ignoring any of your body's fundamental needs or desires? Write about anything else that you noticed. How can you practice giving yourself more of what you need?

Even though your needs may change over time, the fundamentals do not. **Your body needs to breathe and to sleep. She needs food. She needs love. She dies without them.** And there is nothing she must do, no shape or size she must be before she "deserves" food and love and sleep. It's not her fault if she's sick or injured. She's still the astonishing creature she was on the day she was born, a source of joy for those who care about her. **She's yours. She's you.**

We're not suggesting that you "love your body," like that's an easy fix. We're suggesting that you be patient with your body and with your feelings about your body. **Your body is not the enemy.** The real enemy is out there—the Bikini Industrial Complex.

A Note on Physical Activity

When you engage in physical activity, you know it's good for you, because you are 1) completing the cycle and 2) doing a thing.

You also know that most people probably assume you're doing it to "lose weight" or "get in shape," and part of you might still actively want to change the shape of your body. That's all perfectly normal. **Move your body anyway—because it really is good for you—and smile benevolently at the mess.**

Some days it will be messy as hell, other days it will be calm and clear, and every day is just part of the intensely body-neurotic world you happen to live in.

Eating Your Feelings

Burnout is a wound. Wounds need to be cleaned and closed and bandaged so that they can heal properly. And many times, the pain of a wound can cause stress that slows healing, so we need to numb the pain before we do all the other things. The pain of burnout can be numbed by letting your mind escape into comforting books, TV shows, movies, games, etc., and a lot of us also numb our feelings with food. We call this "eating our feelings."

How to Eat Your Feelings (10 min)

Eating your feelings gets vilified because you might *gasp!* consume excess calories. And then you might *gasp!* add fat to your body and become someone who doesn't conform to the socially constructed ideal . . . and, wow, this bag of chips just became a symbol of the white-supremacist patriarchy. But we have a strategy to give you access to this effective numbing strategy that also makes it good for your overall well-being. Here's how.

1. Choose a food based solely on how much you enjoy it. Pleasure is the goal.

   Food:_____

2. Go somewhere comfortable to eat it, and turn attention toward the food.

   a. Use as many senses as you can to appreciate it. Describe the properties of the food—the appearance, flavors, textures, smells.

   b. Describe how the food makes your body feel. This kind of mindful eating can feel refreshing and awakening, or it can reduce an edge of anxiety and allow you to feel more calm and relaxed.

   c. Describe what emotions come up as you experience the food. Does it bring up any special memories of a time or place or person you were with when you previously ate it?

3. For an extra boost, share the experience with someone else.

You Are the New Hotness

When we reconstruct our own standard of beauty with a definition that comes from our own hearts and includes our bodies as they are right now, we can turn toward our bodies with kindness and compassion. Maybe you don't look like you used to, or like you used to imagine you should; but how you look today is the new hotness. It is even better than the old hotness.

- Wearing your new leggings today? You are the new hotness.

- Hair longer or shorter, or a different color or style? New hotness.

- Saggy belly skin from that baby you birthed? New hotness.

- Gained twenty pounds while finishing school? New hotness.

- Skin gets new wrinkles because you lived another year? New hotness.

- Scar tissue following knee-replacement surgery? New hotness.

- Amputation following combat injury? New hotness.

- Mastectomy following breast cancer? New hotness.

The point is, you define and redefine your body's worth, on your own terms. All your body requires of you is that you turn toward it with kindness and compassion, with nonjudgment and plain-vanilla acceptance of all your contradictory emotions, beliefs, and longings. We're not saying that "beautiful" is what your body should be; we're saying beautiful is what your body already is.

New Hotnessing (5 min each, multiple times because this stuff takes practice)

BEGINNER LEVEL: Compliment yourself on your appearance today by writing in the space below. Identify the choices you made about your hair, makeup, clothes, etc. that contribute to how new hotness you are. Did you make some of those choices to help yourself conform to the socially constructed ideal in order to be perceived and accepted more readily? How do you feel about those choices and that acceptance? (5 min)

Bonus: Take a quick picture (without working angles to make yourself look different, just a picture of you as you are) and send it to a friend, saying "new hotness" or whatever phrase communicates to them that you feel like your body is worthy of love just as it is, regardless of the socially constructed ideal.

LEVEL UP: Give your body compliments and write them in the space below. Identify parts of your body you like and what you like about them, just as they are. If you're ready to go hard-core, do this while standing in front of a mirror as close to naked as you comfortably can.

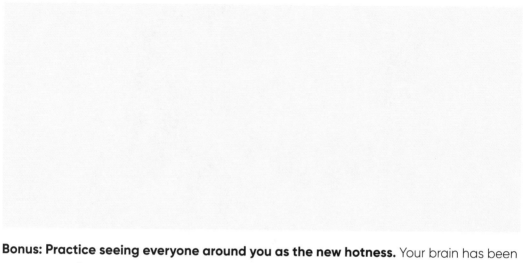

Bonus: Practice seeing everyone around you as the new hotness. Your brain has been programmed to respond to other people's bodies with judgment. When you notice your brain responding to someone's body negatively or positively, remind yourself they're the new hotness. For a catchy tune to remind yourself, see Amelia's "New Hotness Song."

TO WRAP UP THE CHAPTER: Think of some stories, songs, art works, processes, etc. that support or reinforce the ideas in this chapter. (10 min)

OUR EXAMPLES:
Shrill (TV show)
Shrill: Notes from a Loud Woman by Lindy West (book)
The Body Is Not an Apology: The Power of Radical Self-Love
   by Sonya Renee Taylor (book)

YOUR EXAMPLES:

_____

_____

_____

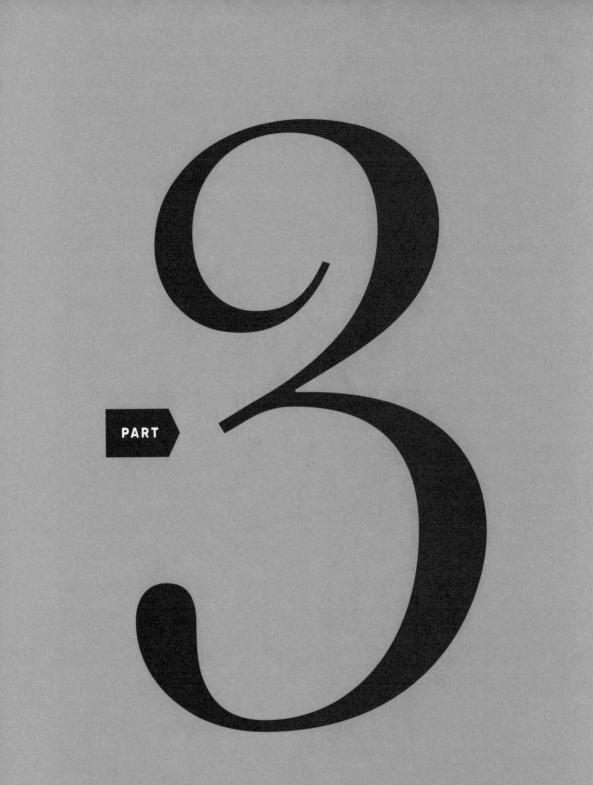

PART 3

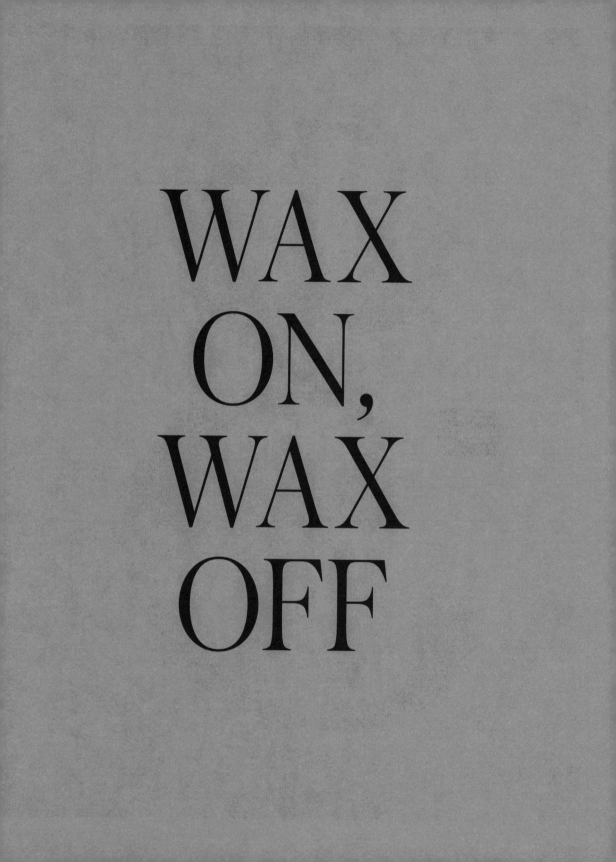

CHAPTER 6

Connect

Reflect Before You Read

It's helpful to notice what preconceptions you have about a topic before learning more about it.

What does "connection" mean to you? Where did you learn what connection was and did that source also teach you the value of connection? Do you have a sense that connection is superior or inferior to autonomy? (5 min)

Social connection is a form of nourishment, like food. Our specific nutritional needs change over the course of our lifespan, but our fundamental need for food does not. Similarly, our specific connectional needs change across our lifespans, but our fundamental need for connection does not.

And, just as we are not built to eat continuously all day every day, we are not meant to be immersed in community all the time. The freedom to oscillate from autonomy to connection is part of the definition of wellness. Unfortunately, the patriarchy values the lone hero over the collective power of many, so we are immersed in messages that stigmatize reaching out for help.

The science disagrees with the patriarchy.

Connection nourishes us in literal, physiological ways, regulating our heart rates and respiration rates, influencing the emotional activations in our brains, shifting our immune responses to injuries and wounds, changing our exposures to stressors, and modulating our stress responses. Simply sharing a physical space with someone—even if they're a stranger—can be enough to coregulate our heartbeats.

Connection is emphatically not just about romantic relationships; it's about having positive relationships of all kinds, including friends, BFFLs, besties, buds, bros, and the fam.

How much connection do you need, and what kind? (20 min)

Turn your attention toward the part of you that connects with others. Does it seem to be longing for more connection? Less? A different kind? Notice if any feelings come up about your need for connection, like pride or shame of autonomy or connection to community.

_____

_____

_____

_____

Try observing those feelings without judgment. Without labeling them "bad" or "good," remember some experiences with connection or autonomy that made you feel refreshed, powerful, and comforted. Then do the same for experiences that exhausted you, left you feeling empty or anxious. What are the differences, and what do they share in common—people, places, species, denomination?

_____

_____

_____

_____

Narrow down the kind of interactions or combination of interactions that feel nurturing for you:

- **Emotional:** not solving a problem, but listening, feeling, and sympathizing together

- **Instrumental:** taking action to help solve a problem

- **Informational:** learning about how to solve a problem

There is no "right amount" of needing to belong; there's just the amount of belonging that feels right for you.

PEOPLE VARY IN THEIR APPETITES FOR CONNECTION. This variability is partly explained by introversion or extroversion, partly by the pleasure an individual experiences in socializing, and partly by a little quirk of personality. Researchers can assess a person's appetite simply by asking whether they agree or disagree with the statement "I have a strong need to belong."

The Bubble of Love

All these energy-creating connections are what we call the "Bubble of Love."

You might experience connection in the Bubble with one person at a time or you might feel it most strongly in large, cooperative groups. You might experience it best with your closest friends. Your spouse. Your church family. Your dog—yes, we experience these kinds of connections with other species, too.

Different Bubbles have different styles; you don't experience or express connection with your Roller Derby teammates the same way you would with your family, and you don't experience or express connection with your family the same way you would with your anti-capitalist, womynist knitting group—but all these different energy-creating Bubbles of Love share two specific ingredients: **trust and connected knowing.**

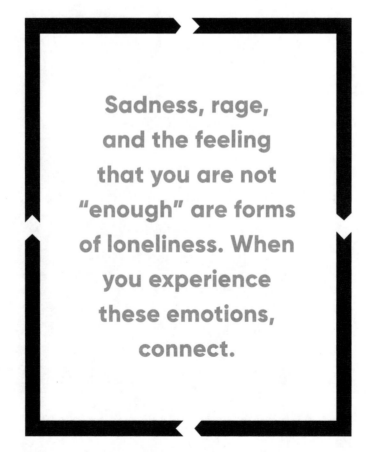

Sadness, rage, and the feeling that you are not "enough" are forms of loneliness. When you experience these emotions, connect.

"What If I Don't Have a Bubble?"

We get this question a lot, and we asked it, too. People assume that, because we're twins, we've also had some special bond, an automatic Bubble. But we grew up in a household with mental illness and addiction, where feelings were silenced and compassion was weakness. By the time we were young adults, we barely spoke to each other. In our late thirties, we started writing *Burnout* together and read all the science that said connection was the cure. Only then did we recognize how drastically our upbringing misled us about connection.

So we started practicing what the research said to do.

Imagine the two of us sitting on opposite sides of a wall, wishing the wall wasn't there, wishing the other person wished the wall wasn't there, ashamed of wishing. Then one day we're reading connection research and one of us says, "Hey, are you over there? Wanna. . . you know. . . smash this damn wall or something?"

The other replies, "Yo, that sounds super awkward and hard. But, yeah, let's try it."

And it was super awkward and hard. We finally talked about the stories we had never talked about. Talked about our feelings, which was very extremely awkward to do when we had been taught that it was forbidden, weak, and dangerous! And we dismantled the wall. It was slow and uncomfortable at first, but the more we did, the easier it got.

The point of this story is to illustrate that you can find connection, because everyone needs connection—including the people around you. They're all longing to connect; but so many of us feel like we have a barrier preventing it. It takes one brave person, empowered by the evidence, to push through the awkward barrier, be the vulnerable one, and connect. You may be surrounded by people who are longing for it just like you are—just like we were—never knowing that they are also surrounded by others who are longing for the same thing. If only one of them knew how simple it was to overcome.

We did it, stilted and fearful as we were taught to be about sharing emotions and being vulnerable. If we can do it, literally anyone can!

Who might you want to be in your Bubble? What can you do to invite them to start connecting more if they feel walled up behind societal expectations to be completely autonomous and independent?

Bubble Ingredient #1: Trust

Lots of species, including humans, keep track of who gives something to another and who reciprocates. The belief that the people around us will reciprocate in proportion to what we give them is called "trust." People who don't trust or who are untrustworthy are energy drains. They belong outside the Bubble.

What we give and receive in relationships can be almost anything—money, time, attention, cupcakes, or compassion for our difficult feelings. That last is the most important of all. If we turn toward someone with our difficult feelings—sadness, anger, hurt—and they tune in to our feelings without judgment or defensiveness, it helps us move through that feeling, like a tunnel, to the light at the end.

This definition of "trust" can be boiled down to one question: "Are you there for me?" Trustworthy people are there for each other, and that mutual trust and trustworthiness maximizes wellness for both people.

Noticing Trust in Your Life (10 min)

Is there now, or has there ever been, someone in your life who you can be "totally yourself" with? Family, friends, a therapist, a colleague, a pet, or a divine presence? In other words, who can you turn to in a difficult time?

_____

_____

_____

_____

How do you feel about that list of those you trust? Do you get the feeling that it "should" be longer? Shorter?

_____

_____

_____

_____

If we insist women "should" develop their identities within the pursuit of "achievement" rather than through relationships, we're pathologizing women's (and every human's) innate search for themselves through connection.

Bubble Ingredient #2: Connected Knowing

Just as the patriarchy respects the lone hero over group work, it prefers understanding that comes intellectually, which means keeping ourselves and our feelings out of it. It's scientific, they say, so it's inherently superior. It's objective, they say, and people's subjective experiences are invalid and unimportant. Facts don't care about your feelings, they say, usually misinterpreting "facts" because they never learned to consider possibilities that are beyond their own experiences.

This "separate" way of knowing is what we're taught in school, and it's a useful way of coming to understand things in certain circumstances. But when we're in the Bubble of Love, we need "connected knowing."

Putting yourself in the shoes of another person to try on their point of view. Temporarily suspending your doubts, judgments, criticisms, and personal needs in favor of exploring someone else's perspective. This is connected knowing.

The most energy-creating characteristic of connected knowing is that it isn't just a way to connect with and understand others, it's a way to connect with and understand our own internal experiences and develop our own identities, through connection with others. Women are more likely to use it than men, if only because women are given greater social permission than men to use their feelings this way. Unfortunately, that's reason enough for the patriarchy to treat it as inferior, unworthy of consideration.

Practicing Connected Knowing (20 min)

BEGINNER LEVEL: Consider a fictional character who is a "villain" in their story. Imagine yourself in their place, with their experiences and their resources. How does that change your thoughts and feelings about that character?

LEVEL UP: Try the same thing for someone with whom you disagree about something subjective, like music or movie preferences. How does it feel to set aside your own, real feelings for a moment in order to understand someone else's?

_____

_____

_____

_____

_____

REAL-LIFE LEVEL: Is there a time when you have set aside your feelings for a moment in a real relationship in order to understand their perspective? What was that like, and what were the results? Have you ever felt like someone was doing this for you? How would it feel to be seen and heard in this way?

_____

_____

_____

_____

_____

ULTRA-MAGE MASTERY LEVEL: Try this exercise with someone on the far opposite end of the political spectrum from you. How does it feel to consider this possibility? When might it be worthwhile to try?

_____

_____

_____

_____

_____

Signs You Need to Recharge in the Bubble of Love

Here we'll describe four signs that you need to disengage from your autonomous efforts and seek connections with others. Each of these experiences is a different form of hunger for connection—that is, they're all different ways of feeling lonely. Take note of any that ring true for you, and what sort of connection would help in the circumstance.

1. **WHEN YOU HAVE BEEN GASLIT.** When you're asking yourself, "Am I crazy, or is something completely unacceptable happening right now?" turn to someone who can relate; let them give you the reality check that yes, the gaslights are flickering.

2. **WHEN YOU FEEL "NOT ENOUGH."** When you experience the empty-handed feeling that you are just one person, unable to meet all the demands the world makes on you, helpless in the face of the endless, yawning need you see around you, recognize that emotion for what it is: a form of loneliness.

3. **WHEN YOU'RE SAD.** Many of us have been taught to keep our sadness under control because it makes others uncomfortable. But we find our way out of that tunnel most efficiently when we have a friend who calls through the darkness to say, "I'm right here!" Or better yet, when someone can take our hand in the dark and say, "Any step we take together is a step toward the light."

4. **WHEN YOU ARE BOILING WITH RAGE.** Many of us have been taught to swallow our rage, to hide it even from ourselves (and more than our sadness). Rage gives you strength and energy and the urge to fight, and sharing that energy in the Bubble changes it from something potentially dangerous to something safe and potentially transformative.

Recognizing Your Bubble (5min)

Recall a time when your Bubble showed up for you. What were you going through? Who showed up for you? What did they do for you? Have you given similar support to them?

Über-Bubble *or* How to Connect When You Need to Recharge *or* How to Complete the Cycle While Connecting

Über-bubble is a magic trick. It's a special combination for the most stress-relieving, refueling experiences of a person's life. The combo is this: moving together toward a shared purpose. That means, for maximum impact, get yourself in physical proximity to other people and move your bodies with a shared intention.

This combination not only offers an intense, stress-relieving experience, but it also gives humans access to an elevated, uplifted feeling like they are one with the universe, like their individuality opens a door to a greater collective power.

Here are some examples:

- Go dancing, or better yet, attend a festival where everyone is immersed in music and fandom.

- Worship with others, especially if the service takes place in an inspiring location.

- March in a protest to protect the rights of the disenfranchised.

What's your über-bubble? What experiences have made you feel part of something greater, connected, and uplifted? Describe the circumstances—people, places, things, sounds, smells, sights—and the feelings. How long did the feeling impact you? Does recalling it now change how you feel in this moment? (10 min)

TO WRAP UP THE CHAPTER: Think of some stories, songs, art works, processes, etc. that support or reinforce the ideas in this chapter. (10 min)

OUR EXAMPLES:
Frozen (movie)
Hair Love (movie)

YOUR EXAMPLES:

CHAPTER 7

What Makes You Stronger

Reflect Before You Read

It's helpful to notice what preconceptions you have about a topic before learning more about it.

What does the word "rest" mean to you? Has it ever meant something different? Where did you learn how much rest you need? What would it mean if your need for rest suddenly increased or decreased? Does there seem to be a moral or ethical connotation to rest? (5 min)

_____

_____

_____

_____

What makes you stronger is rest. "Rest" doesn't just mean sleep—though, of course, sleep is essential. Rest also includes switching from one type of activity to another, when you stop using a part of you that's worn out, damaged, or inflamed, so that it has a chance to renew itself.

Mental energy, like stress, has a cycle it runs through. We oscillate from focus to processing and back to focus. The idea that you can use "grit" or "self-control" to stay focused and productive every minute of every day is not merely incorrect, it is gaslighting, and it is potentially damaging to your brain.

Life in the modern developed world is such that many of us have a vast overabundance of virtually everything . . . yet often we can't meet our basic, life-sustaining, physiological needs without feeling guilty, ashamed, lazy, greedy, conflicted, or, at best, defiant. As "human givers," women live with the expectation that we give every part of our humanity, including our bodies, our health, and our very lives. Our time, energy, and attention should go toward someone else's well-being, not be squandered on our own.

But we are built to oscillate between work and rest. When we allow for this oscillation, the quality of our work improves, along with our health. Rest makes us more persistent and productive. More importantly, it allows us to feel our best, and to be our best selves.

Sleep

Since *Burnout* was released, we have spoken to thousands more women about their stress. We have heard dozens of their stories, and answered hundreds of their questions.

Most of their questions were about sleep.

And that makes sense. Everything from physical activity to learning to emotions are integrated and strengthened while you sleep. Your bones, blood vessels, digestive system, muscles (including your heart), and all your other body tissues heal from the damage you inflicted on them during the day. Your memories consolidate and new information is integrated into existing knowledge. You can dream about beating the daylights out of your enemy, and you'll wake up feeling released from the grip of your rage, better able to handle interpersonal conflict.

This is not an area of research where there's any reasonable debate. The medical opinion is in: Sleep is good for you, and not sleeping is bad for you in every way—dangerous and potentially lethal. **If you make only one change in your life after reading this book, let it be getting more sleep.**

So, this is the longest chapter, and it goes into the most detail. Let's start with sleep 101, then move on to the different factors that vary with every individual.

Where to start to get your best sleep:

1. Manage your environment. It is possible to adapt to pretty much any environment, but **for most people, an ideal sleep environment is a) cool, b) dark, and c) quiet**. Try adding more of those things to your space for a week or two and see if it helps.

    a. If you can't cool down the room, you can trick your body into cooling down by taking a hot bath or shower before bed. After your body temperature is artificially raised, the drop back to normal mimics the cooling that happens as you fall asleep.

b. Blue and cool white lights are the most likely to interfere with sleep. You might find a warm light comforting in the dark, or you may need total darkness. If you can't darken a room completely, sleep masks are another option. For those who have a strong sensory response to masks, there are designs that are tight, loose, thick and padded, thin and flexible. Or you can wear a nightcap and pull it down over your eyes.

c. Some minds just don't settle in the quiet. That's normal, too. Try adding various types of white noise, music that allows your brain to turn off, or even a familiar audiobook—it's not just kids who like being read to sleep. Devices and apps these days have sleep modes and timers designed for exactly this purpose.

2. Keep a routine. Most people thrive on a consistent sleep schedule—we'll talk about all the variables in detail below, but whatever you discover works best for you, your body will like it if you can keep it predictable and regular. A presleep routine also helps teach your body when to kick into sleepy-time mode.

3. Remember that any sleep advice you read is generalized, and not all of it will apply to you. Articles are published every day that insist there's an ideal way to sleep, or certain kinds of sleep are linked with certain diseases. There is zero research that applies to everyone, and any research that's new is basically just a suggestion to other scientists that there's an interesting question to probe further. Journalists and "body hackers" will try to make it sound like scientists know exactly how you should sleep, but only your body can tell you what kind of sleep you need.

Let's look at some of the factors that vary from person to person.

Quantity and Quality

The cure for being tired is getting more sleep. And it's pretty much the only cure. There's no hack for teaching your body to survive on less sleep. Most of us need between seven and nine hours of sleep in every twenty-four-hour period. The quantity of sleep you need changes over your lifetime—you need way more when you're an infant than you do as an adult, and adolescents (from about age fourteen to twenty-five) need more sleep than their parents. There are rare outliers who need more or less, but the point is to sleep until you feel rested. If you are sleeping more than nine hours a night and *still don't feel rested*, go see a medical professional. Otherwise, there is nothing better or worse about being a seven-and-one-half-hour sleeper like Emily, or a nine-hour sleeper like Amelia.

Recognizing the Moral Value Imposed on Sleep (10 min)

Pretend this is a social media post from a rich and famous actress with millions of followers:

😲, y'all.

I've been sleeping 9 or 10 hours

every night for the past month!

What would some of the comments be?

_____

_____

_____

Now pretend this was her social media post:

😲, y'all.

I've been sleeping 5 or 6 hours

every night for the past month!

What would some of the comments be?

_____

_____

_____

How many of these various perspectives have made their way into your expectations about how much you should sleep? What about how much your loved ones should sleep?

_____

_____

_____

If you're not sure what quantity of sleep you need, it can be tricky to find out while also participating in the rush of life that overwhelms so many of us. The most efficient way to find out is simply to track your sleep and how rested you feel, and discover how much sleep it takes for you to feel your best. Be aware that, when you believe you're "almost asleep," you're probably already asleep, so you may be getting more sleep than you know. A rough idea is all you'll need to make tracking helpful.

Tracking Your Sleep and Mood (5 min per day for one week)

Here's a simple chart to track the number of hours you sleep, and also your overall feeling of being well rested on a scale of 1 to 10. Pick one color for sleep and another for rest and mark each one each day.

DATE	HOURS OF SLEEP												ENERGY LEVEL		
DAY	1	2	3	4	5	6	7	8	9	10	11	12	– MINIMUM / MAXIMUM +		

Chronotype (aka Early Bird vs. Night Owl)

Everybody has a built-in schedule that changes gradually with age. You may already know what works for you, but if your schedule has always been dictated by external forces, like school and work, you may not be sure.

Identifying Your Chronotype (10 min)

If we told you that you had to stay up late every night this week, how would that feel?

_____

_____

_____

If we told you that you had to get up early every morning this week, how would that feel?

_____

_____

_____

When you're on vacation and you don't have to conform to a schedule, how does your sleep schedule change? Have you experienced a schedule that you wished you could keep up?

_____

_____

_____

Chronotype is not black or white, early or late. And it doesn't stay stable your whole life. It's complicated. What conclusions do these reflections guide you toward?

_____

_____

_____

Segmentation

Some folks need one long night's sleep—they are monophasic sleepers. Many folks wake up for an hour or two in the middle of the night, then fall back asleep. Others do better with a shorter night's sleep and a long nap during the day.

As with the other variables, there's no "better" or "worse" way to sleep—the point is to discover how your body sleeps best, and discover if you can use that knowledge to improve your well-being.

What kind of sleep segmentation works for you? Choose your answer to the following questions. Feel free to note details if the answer requires more nuance. (5 min)

- Do you often wake in the middle of the night? **yes** or **no**

- If you wake in the middle of the night, do you generally fall back asleep without effort? **yes** or **no**

- Do naps help you? **yes** or **no**

- When you imagine examples of sleep segmentation, is your impression of them negative or positive? **negative** or **positive**

- Do they feel like weird interruptions to otherwise good sleep, or might they be healthy segments within a larger cycle of good sleep? **weird interruptions** or **healthy segments**

If your schedule didn't dictate your sleep schedule, what kind of segmentation would feel comfortable for you?

_____

_____

_____

_____

_____

A Note About Naps

If you wake up from a nap and feel less rested, there are a few possible reasons.

1. You may not be a napper. Almost half of people just aren't. That's normal.

2. You took the wrong length nap. Sleep (like everything your body does) happens in cycles, and a nap won't feel restful if you wake to an alarm in the middle of the cycle. Ideally, you'll fall asleep and wake up spontaneously, but if you have to stick to a schedule, try twenty minutes instead of an hour so you're less likely to interrupt a cycle.

3. You're extremely sleep deprived. When our bodies haven't had enough sleep, they compensate by pumping us full of adrenaline and other hormones to allow us to cope until we can pay off our sleep debt. After a nap, your body is slightly more rested, so it doesn't need to compensate anymore. The result is you are more rested, but you feel your fatigue more than you did before.

Daydreaming

Sleep is a twenty-four-hour cycle, but our brains need rest at shorter intervals, too. When you allow your brain to oscillate from intentional focus to free wandering, your work improves as well as your health.

When you drop out of task-focused attention and into neutral, your "resting" brain is not doing nothing—far from it. Running in the background of your awareness is what neuroscientists call the "default mode network," a collection of linked brain areas that function as a kind of low-grade dreaming. It feels like your mind is wandering, but your brain is actually assessing the present state and planning for the future—like a chess-playing computer rapidly scanning the board and running simulations.

Mental rest is not idleness. It is the time necessary for your brain to process the world. If you've ever had an epiphany in the shower, you can thank the default mode network.

Practice Daydreaming (3 min)

Trace the circle pattern below, or color it in, or do something else that will keep your hands busy but that requires no mental focus. Brushing your teeth is good for this. Most important: Make the choice to spend this time doing nothing else, and don't try to accomplish anything or to maintain focus on your breathing or anything else. Ideally, keep going until your brain brings itself back.

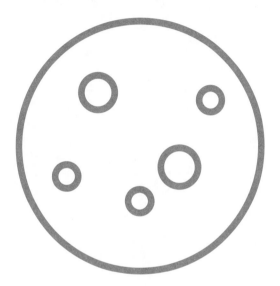

When you brought your attention back, did you feel at all rested or refreshed, or more ready to move forward than you were before? Have you had that experience in the past, or have you felt guilty for letting your mind wander?

_____

_____

_____

_____

_____

_____

_____

_____

The number one cause of insomnia is worry about sleep. So, if you're lying awake, staring at the clock and counting hours, reduce your worry by remembering that just lying there, giving your body a chance to rest, is valuable. You're doing your best, and that's enough.

Active Rest

If daydreaming feels painfully boring to you, good news! "Active rest" is an important way to access rest even if it does sound oxymoronic. You do it by shifting gears, so that you rest the one you've been using, and go into another one instead. The task you switch to doesn't have to be a low-demand task, it can be another kind of work. For example, shift from reading to cleaning, from cleaning to doing your hair. Or, like Emily, shift from writing a self-help book to writing a romance novel. Or, like Rachel Maddow, shift from analyzing current events to chopping wood.

Discovering Your Effective Active Rest (5 min)

Think about the demanding tasks in your life, and what activity might be a refreshing change, even if it seems like it might be more work.

When I'm _____,

it feels refreshing to switch to _____.

When I'm _____,

it feels refreshing to switch to _____.

When I'm _____, .

it feels refreshing to switch to _____.

So, How Much Rest Is "Adequate"?

Science says 42 percent.

That's the percentage of time your body and brain need you to spend resting, including sleep. It's about ten hours out of every twenty-four. It doesn't have to be every day; it can average out over a week or a month or more. But yeah. That much.

We're not saying you *should* take 42 percent of your time to rest; we're saying if you don't take the 42 percent, the 42 percent *will take you*. Our biology requires that we spend 42 percent of our lives maintaining the organism of our physical existence.

Here's what your 42 percent might look like:

These are just averages, and as you can see, you'll sometimes do more than one thing at a time. Some people need more sleep than others. Natural exercisers may want to spend more time on physical activity. Foodies may want to spend more time on food. Extroverts may want to spend as much of this time as possible with other people. Your mileage may vary; fine-tune it to fit your individual needs.

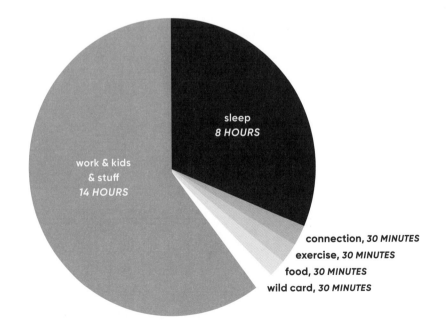

sleep
8 HOURS

work & kids
& stuff
14 HOURS

connection, *30 MINUTES*
exercise, *30 MINUTES*
food, *30 MINUTES*
wild card, *30 MINUTES*

- Eight hours of sleep opportunity, give or take an hour.

- Twenty to thirty minutes of "stress-reducing conversation" with your partner or other trusted loved one.

- Thirty minutes of physical activity. Whether with people or alone, you do it with the explicit mindset of gear-switching, Feels-purging, rest-getting freedom. Physical activity counts as "rest" partly because it improves the quality of your sleep and partly because it completes the stress response cycle, transitioning your body out of a stressed state and into a resting state.

- Thirty minutes of paying attention to food. "Thirty minutes?" you say. Don't fret. That includes all meals, shopping, cooking, and eating, and it doesn't have to be all at once. It can be with people or alone, but it can't be while working or driving or watching TV or even listening to a podcast. Pay attention to your food for half an hour a day. This counts as rest partly because it provides necessary nourishment and partly because it's active rest, a change of pace, apart from the other domains of your life. Think of it as meditation.

- And a thirty-minute wild card, depending on your needs. For some people, this will be extra physical activity, because they need that much to feel good. For others, it will be preparation for their sleep opportunity, because they know their brains need time to transition from the buzzing state of wakefulness into the quiet that allows the brain to sleep. For still others, it will be social play time, because their appetite for social engagement is strong. And for some, it's simply a buffer for travel and changing clothes and other rest-preparation time (because: reality) during which you engage your default mode network—that is, you let your mind wander.

Now let's actually track how you spend your hours, then you can chart your actual percentages. Turn to the next page to fill out the pie chart and then begin completing the 24/7 Worksheet that starts on page 128.

Where Can You Find the Time? (20 min)

Fill out the pie chart below based on how much time on average you estimate you spend on each category per day (make sure your time spent totals twenty-four hours and feel free to omit a category if it doesn't apply):

-**Work & Commute**
-**Sleep**
-**Leisure & Sport**
-**Eating**
-**Household Chores**
-**Caring for Others**
-**Other**

Broken down this way, it's almost painfully simple and obvious: sleep, food, friends, and movement.

Are there any surprises about the chart you filled out? How might you increase your rest going forward?

_____

_____

If you're thinking, "I can get by with less," you're right. You can "get by," dragging your increasingly rest-deprived brain and body through your life. But no one who cares about your well-being will expect you to sustain that way of life for an extended period of time. No one in your Bubble of Love wants you to "get by"; they want you to thrive and grow stronger. We want you to thrive and grow stronger. What makes you stronger is rest.

24/7 Worksheet (40 min)

You can use the worksheets on the following pages to track your time and notice the opportunities you can create to increase the rest you're getting. On the first calendar, mark your actual time use. If you have a pretty stable schedule, you can fill it out all at once. If your schedule tends to change, fill it out each day to see how these next seven days go.

1. Block out time for sleep. *At minimum,* it should be a realistic representation of when you really do sleep. Be sure to include in your sleep time how long it takes you to fall asleep and the time between when your alarm goes off and when you actually get up. This is your complete "sleep opportunity."

2. Block out regularly occurring events, including:

a. work (with commute);

b. kids' activities and care;

c. social activities, including those with partner (don't forget sex);

d. meals, including preparation time;

e. bathing/showering/hair time;

f. shopping (including groceries and online shopping); and

g. TV, internet/social media use, solo games, and staring at your phone.

3. Approximate less regular but anticipatable activities, like doctors' appointments, car maintenance, home repair, etc. A simple way to get a rough estimate is to look at how much time you've spent on these things over the previous twelve months. Add up all that time, divide it by fifty-two, and you'll have the average time per week.

4. Color code each activity by types of needs they fulfill: connection, rest (both sleep and mind wandering), meaning, and completing the cycle.

On the second calendar ("Ideal" 24/7 Calendar), imagine the ways you might, hypothetically, make your time use more like the "ideal"—"ideal" being entirely subjective. You're the one who knows whether you need more sleep, more stress-cycle completion, more connection, or just more time.

1. Ideally, your sleep schedule is a solid block of the same seven to nine hours every day, including weekends, but you can make up a shortfall with naps or extra sleep on the weekends.

2. Reserve thirty minutes of each day for a "stress-reducing conversation." If your stress-reducing conversation partner is your life partner, you might also add a weekly hour-long "state of the union" conversation. Research recommends these as the standards for sustaining a satisfying relationship.

3. Include thirty to sixty minutes for physical activity three to six days per week, plus any prep/travel time.

4. Code as before—social, rest, meaning, and completing the cycle.

5. Code some activities, like some phone use, shopping, or meal prep that you haven't been using for mind-wandering rest time, and see if you can transition your state of mind from one of fretful worry to calm future-mapping.

6. **BONUS:** Mark activities that smash patriarchy. Examples: If you work in a job where women are underrepresented, all your work and commute time is patriarchy smashin'. If you parent a child with the goal of transmitting positive and inclusive gender norms, that's patriarchy smashin'. If you are a woman of color, a hijabi in the West, not heterosexual or cisgender, or live with a disability or chronic illness, etc., literally every moment is patriarchy smashin'. Remember that "Joy is an act of resistance," (Toi Derricote) and "Rest is resistance," (Tricia Hersey). Any time you remember you deserve resources like pleasure and rest and care, you defy the narrative of Human Giver Syndrome, and you smash!

	SUNDAY	MONDAY	TUESDAY	
6 A.M.				
7 A.M.				
8 A.M.				
9 A.M.				
10 A.M.				
11 A.M.				
NOON				
1 P.M.				
2 P.M.				
3 P.M.				
4 P.M.				
5 P.M.				
6 P.M.				
7 P.M.				
8 P.M.				
9 P.M.				
10 P.M.				
11 P.M.				
12 A.M.				
1 A.M.				
2 A.M.				
3 A.M.				
4 A.M.				
5 A.M.				

WEDNESDAY	THURSDAY	FRIDAY	SATURDAY

	SUNDAY	MONDAY	TUESDAY	
6 A.M.				
7 A.M.				
8 A.M.				
9 A.M.				
10 A.M.				
11 A.M.				
NOON				
1 P.M.				
2 P.M.				
3 P.M.				
4 P.M.				
5 P.M.				
6 P.M.				
7 P.M.				
8 P.M.				
9 P.M.				
10 P.M.				
11 P.M.				
12 A.M.				
1 A.M.				
2 A.M.				
3 A.M.				
4 A.M.				
5 A.M.				

WEDNESDAY	THURSDAY	FRIDAY	SATURDAY

The payoff of spending more time resting is that during the remaining 58 percent of your life, you're more energized, more focused, more creative, and nicer to be around—not to mention a safer driver, less likely to make mistakes that will cost you later, and more likely to enjoy what you're doing, rather than simply feeling that it's the "right" thing to do.

The Slow Leak

Judging your need for rest is a slow leak that drains the effectiveness of the rest you get. We've established that rest is what makes you stronger, and we already know Human Giver Syndrome doesn't want you to be stronger. But we want you to be strong, healthy, confident, and joyful, so it's time to turn toward those slow leaks and patch them with kindness and compassion.

Plugging the Slow Leak (5 min)

Reflect on moments when you've felt guilty for sleeping, or you've thought you might be "lazy" because you wanted a break.

Where did those judgmental ideas come from? Where did you learn them and from whom?

_____

_____

_____

_____

_____

_____

Imagine a friend tells you she feels guilty for sleeping or lazy for wanting a break. What would you tell her? Does she deserve rest?

_____

_____

_____

_____

_____

_____

TO WRAP UP THE CHAPTER: Think of some stories, songs, art works, processes, etc. that support or reinforce the ideas in this chapter. (10 min)

OUR EXAMPLES:

The Sims 4 (video game)

The Nap Ministry by Tricia Hersey (social media channel)

Rest Is Resistance: A Manifesto by Tricia Hersey (book)

YOUR EXAMPLES:

Rest matters because you matter. You are not here to be "productive." You are here to be you, to engage with your Something Larger, to move through the world with confidence and joy. And to do that, you require rest.

CHAPTER 8

Grow Mighty

Reflect Before You Read

It's helpful to notice what preconceptions you have about a topic before learning more about it.

What does "self-compassion" mean to you? What does "self-criticism" mean? Where did you first learn about them, and in what ways have those first lessons stayed with you or changed you? (5 min)

You deserve respect and love; you deserve to be cherished. You deserve kindness, right now, just as you are. Not when you lose ten pounds, or a hundred. Not when you get a promotion or finish your degree or get married or come out or have a baby. Now.

The Madwoman in the Attic

Sometimes we fall short of what the world expects of us—whether those expectations were explicit or just implied. And sometimes we're the ones who decide whether our bodies know this is dangerous. Folks who exist on the fringes because they don't conform to the socially constructed ideal are in danger when the lion comes. Wanting to fit in isn't a petty or trite desire that can just be ignored; it's part of our evolutionary heritage.

As a result, most of us have a mean stranger in our head who is beating us up, pushing us unrelentingly toward conforming. We'll call her "the Madwoman in the Attic," following a literary trope from Charlotte Brontë's *Jane Eyre*. In that story, one of the main characters keeps a madwoman locked away in his attic. And, like, don't we all? She's that voice of self-criticism that tells us we're not good enough, that we're failures or imposters, and that we are broken and undeserving.

We use the term *madwoman* advisedly, as women with chronic mental illnesses of our own, not to mock or dismiss the experience of the Madwoman, but to empathize with her experience. This uncomfortable, fragile part of ourselves serves a very important function. She grew inside us, to manage the chasm between who we are and who Human Giver Syndrome expects us to be. She is the part of us that has the impossible, tormenting task of bridging the unbridgeable chasm between us and this "expected-us." When that chasm looms, our madwoman assesses the situation and decides what the problem is. She has only two options: The world is a lying asshole with bogus expectations. Or there is something wrong with *us*.

Some madwomen are more protective than destructive; some are more sad than angry; some have a sense of humor. They are the shadow, the hurt little girl, the downtrodden teenager, the "perfect" version of ourselves, the crazy lady in the attic yelling terrible things that echo through the house.

Every madwoman is just trying to keep us safe. But her task is impossible—none of us will ever be what the world expects, because those expectations are contradictory and impossible. And an impossible task will make anyone more angry and mean, while underneath they're just exhausted and hurt and scared.

Your madwoman might look like anything, if she has a visible form at all. Emily's madwoman looks like Te Kā, the lava monster from *Moana*. Amelia's looks like this.

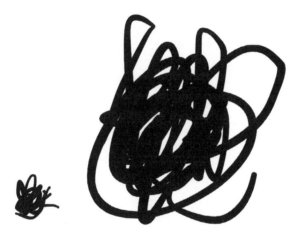

Tune in to the discomfort you feel when you fail to conform to who the world expects you to be, when you feel like you've failed or are an imposter. It may help to recall a time when you felt shame or guilt for falling short of expectations, then turn your attention to the feeling itself and examine it without evaluating it as good or bad.

Many of us perceive that feeling coming from a person in your imagination. What does she look like, or how do you perceive her? If her appearance isn't person-like, it might be a shape or shadow or light; or you might perceive her as a physical sensation or disembodied voice. However she comes to you, describe all the details you notice.

Get to Know Your Madwoman (40 min)

What is your madwoman like? Take a few minutes to imagine her—both her uncomfortableness and her fragility. Describe her in words. Sketch her.

When was she born? What is her history? What does she say to you?

Write out her feelings and thoughts. Notice where she's harshly critical of you, shaming, or perfectionistic. You may even want to mark those places. Highlight them in different colors. Those are sources of exhaustion. Can you hear sadness or fear under her madness?

Ask her what she fears or what she's grieving. Listen to her stories—never forgetting that she's a madwoman. Remind her that you are the grown-up, the homeowner, or the teacher, and she can trust you to maintain the attic so that she always has a safe place to stay.

Thank her for the hard work she has done to help you survive.

Befriend Your Madwoman

Turn toward your madwoman with curiosity. Ask her some questions.

What does your madwoman say about you? What does she say about the expectations the world has for you?

_____

_____

_____

_____

_____

After she expresses her criticism and anger, what do you hear is motivating her frustration? Fear? Loneliness? Despair?

_____

_____

_____

_____

_____

Turn toward that self-critical part of you with kindness and compassion. Write a short note of understanding and compassion below.

_____

_____

_____

_____

_____

A Note on Perfectionism

These days, "I'm a perfectionist" is used casually as a kind of humble brag, but let's be clear about how perfectionism can serve as a generally benign or a potentially harmful manifestation of the madwoman.

- **Generally benign:** preferring tidiness and organization over messiness; being detail-oriented and checking your work for mistakes; and having high standards for yourself or others.

- **Generally toxic:** believing that if things aren't perfect, they aren't any good (e.g., if you make one mistake, everything is ruined), and feeling pressure from other people to succeed at everything you do. These domains of perfectionism are associated with depression, anxiety, disordered eating, negative relationships, and feelings of helplessness in the world.

The fundamental problem with perfectionism is that it does terrible things to your Monitor. You have the goal of "perfection," which is an impossible goal, as you start the project or the meal or the outfit or the day, and then as soon as something falls short of "perfect," the whole thing is ruined. And sometimes if your goal is "perfect," some part of you already knows that it's an impossible goal, so you think about your project or meal or outfit or day, knowing you're never going to achieve your goal, and so you feel hopeless before you even begin.

Self-Compassion

The purpose of personifying your madwoman is to separate yourself from her, to create a dynamic where you can relate to her the way you relate to your friends—with connected knowing. When we can personify our self-criticism, we can relate to it more effectively. We can build a relationship with our madwoman—maybe even a friendship.

This is self-compassion. There is a popular notion that we should ignore the negative voices in our head and brush away self-doubt. But that voice is coming from a real place inside you, and ignoring it willl bury that place, not help it become safer and more healing.

During the last twenty years there has been an explosion of research that shows us how much better people do when they engage in less self-criticism and more self-compassion. Self-compassion reduces depression, anxiety, and disordered eating. It improves overall life satisfaction. When you are gentle with yourself, you grow mighty.

Diligent practice of self-compassion works; it lowers stress hormones and improves mood. And many years of research have confirmed that self-forgiveness is associated with greater physical and mental well-being—all without diminishing your motivation to do the things that matter to you.

When you're seriously struggling, and positive reappraisal isn't enough to make the struggle tolerable, self-compassion can help. Turning toward your internal experience with kindness and compassion is more healing than positive reappraisal.

Recognizing Why Self-Compassion Is Hard

1. We feel the need to beat ourselves up in order to grow.

You've been listening to the madwoman, hurting from her insults for most of your life. And you're still here, having accomplished a bunch of things! So, you start to believe that the suffering is why you achieved. You worry that if you start practicing compassion, you'll stop growing and progressing.

But is there anything that grows and thrives if you punish it constantly? Nope. Everything thrives best when it is loved and nurtured. Including you.

If it still feels dangerous to let go of harsh self-criticism, start by practicing compassion toward others, which comes more easily to many of us.

Loving-kindness Meditation (10 min)

1. Get into a comfortable position, and decide to focus your mind on loving-kindness.

2. Think of someone you love. Write down their name and what they mean to you.

Now, in your mind, wish them love, compassion, peace, and ease.

3. Think of someone you are acquainted with, but not close to. Write down their name and what makes them so memorable.

Now, in your mind, wish them love, compassion, peace, and ease.

4. Think of a stranger you've never spoken with. Write down where you saw them.

Now, in your mind, wish them love, compassion, peace, and ease.

5. If you'd like to go even deeper and learn how far loving-kindness can go, imagine someone you dislike. Try to identify someone who displays their humanity and write down their name. Can you imagine them eating? Going to the bathroom?

_____

_____

Now, in your mind, wish them love, compassion, peace, and ease.

6. If you're interested in going further, you could imagine a person who you might even call an enemy. Who are they? What do they mean to you?

_____

_____

Now, in your mind, wish them love, compassion, peace, and ease.

7. Okay, maybe this one is the hardest. Imagine yourself. What feelings surface first about yourself and your humanity?

_____

_____

Now, in your mind, wish yourself love, compassion, peace, and ease.

2. Healing hurts.

Once you stop reopening wounds you've been inflicting on yourself for years, they finally begin to heal. And this healing creates a new kind of pain—one that can't be managed by the same strategies you've been using to manage the pain of the whip. You were good at managing that old kind of pain, and now you have to learn a whole new way to deal with this whole new kind of pain.

As a sunburn heals, you have to learn to deal with the itching. As a limb heals, you have to manage the discomfort of physical therapy. And as emotional wounds heal, there are mental consequences that need to be acknowledged and treated. Here are some ways to do that:

1. Speak to someone in your Bubble about it or a professional therapist.

2. If you feel like you've been on an endless slog, recognize the change, growth, and progress you've made. Find the wins you've had so far (chapter 2).

3. Complete the stress cycles initiated by this process.

4. Revisit the most helpful exercises in this workbook to remind yourself that it's worth the work.

3. Strength is scary.

The truth is that a lot of us fear how mighty we could grow if we were no longer draining our energy by managing all the self-inflicted pain of self-criticism.

We know that with greater personal power would come greater personal responsibilities, and we're afraid that when we have the greater power, we won't be able to deal with those greater responsibilities.

The difficulty of imagining ourselves with the knowledge, expertise, and strength we will gain in the future can stop us entirely from moving toward that future.

Imagine a future without the pain and stress of self-criticism. How do you feel about the idea of being that strong? What does this version of yourself look and feel like?

Everyone's life is different, and we are all doing our best. "Our best" today may not be "the best there is," but it's the best we can do today. Which is strange. And yet true. And this truth could draw us down into feelings of helplessness and isolation if we don't stay anchored. And the way we stay anchored is with gratitude.

Gratitude

It's not a self-help book for women without the injunction to "practice gratitude," right? Gratitude practices really are good for you, but before we discuss them, let's mention one caveat: Being grateful for good things doesn't erase the difficult things.

For centuries, women have been told to be grateful for how much better we have it now than we did before. This "gratitude for what we have" has been used as a weapon against us, to silence our struggle and shame us for our suffering. Gratitude is not about ignoring problems. If anything, gratitude works by providing tools for the struggle, for further progress. It is positive reappraisal, concentrated and distilled to its purest essence. And forgetting to be grateful is completely normal, which is why we all need to be reminded.

So, how do we do it?

The key is practicing gratitude-for-who-you-have and gratitude-for-how-things-happen.

Gratitude-for-Who-You-Have (30 min)

Mr. Rogers, accepting a Lifetime Achievement Award, asked everyone in the audience to take ten seconds to remember some of the people who have "helped you love the good that grows within you, some of those people who have loved us and wanted what was best for us, [. . .] those who have encouraged us to become who we are."

Give it a try for a short-term quick-fix gratitude boost. Follow Mr. Rogers's instructions now. Write what came to mind below.

Now, write that person a letter expressing how they helped you.

Dear _____,

_____

_____

_____

_____

_____

_____

_____

_____

_____

_____

_____

_____

_____

_____

_____

_____

_____

Love, _____

When you're finished, you may even want to give it to them. Better still, read the letter out loud to them. A "gratitude visit" like this can boost your well-being for a full month, or even up to three months.

Gratitude-for-How-Things-Happen (10 min per day for a week)

This is an exercise for a longer-term gratitude lift. At the end of each day, think of some event or circumstance for which you feel grateful, and write about it. It will train your brain to notice not just the positive events themselves, but also the personal strengths you leveraged to create them and the external resources that made them possible.

- Give the event or circumstance a title, like "Finished Writing Chapter 8" or "Made It Through That Meeting Without Crying or Yelling."

- Write down what happened, including details about what anyone involved, including you, did or said.

- Describe how it made you feel at the time, and how you feel now, as you think about it.

- Explain how the event or circumstance came to be. What was the cause? What confluence of circumstances came together to create this moment?

If, as you write, you feel yourself being drawn into negative, critical thoughts and feelings, gently set them to one side and return your attention to the thing you're being grateful for.

We recommend trying this exercise for one event per day for three weeks. If you're feeling super ambitious, try it for three events every day, for at least a week.

To start, try keeping a gratitude journal for a week, using the following pages.

Title: _____

_____

What happened: _____

_____

_____

_____

_____

_____

How you felt, then and now: _____

_____

_____

_____

_____

How it came to be: _____

_____

_____

_____

_____

_____

Title: _____

_____

What happened: _____

_____

_____

_____

_____

_____

_____

How you felt, then and now: _____

_____

_____

_____

_____

_____

_____

_____

How it came to be: _____

_____

_____

_____

_____

_____

_____

Title:_____

_____

What happened:_____

_____

_____

_____

_____

_____

_____

How you felt, then and now:_____

_____

_____

_____

_____

_____

_____

_____

How it came to be:_____

_____

_____

_____

_____

_____

_____

Title: _____

_____

What happened: _____

_____

_____

_____

_____

_____

_____

_____

How you felt, then and now: _____

_____

_____

_____

_____

_____

_____

_____

How it came to be: _____

_____

_____

_____

_____

_____

_____

_____

Title: _____

_____

What happened: _____

_____

_____

_____

_____

_____

_____

How you felt, then and now: _____

_____

_____

_____

_____

_____

_____

How it came to be: _____

_____

_____

_____

_____

_____

_____

_____

Title:_____

_____

What happened:_____

_____

_____

_____

_____

_____

_____

How you felt, then and now:_____

_____

_____

_____

_____

_____

_____

How it came to be:_____

_____

_____

_____

_____

_____

_____

Title: _____

_____

What happened: _____

_____

_____

_____

_____

_____

_____

How you felt, then and now: _____

_____

_____

_____

_____

_____

_____

How it came to be: _____

_____

_____

_____

_____

_____

_____

The world does not have to change before we turn toward our internal experiences with kindness and compassion. And when we do, that, all by itself, is a revolution. The world is changed when we change, because we—each of us (and that includes you)—are a part of the world. This is our shared home, and we, Emily and Amelia, are your sisters.

TO WRAP UP THE CHAPTER: Think of some stories, songs, art works, processes, etc. that support or reinforce the ideas in this chapter. (10 min)

OUR EXAMPLES:
Jane Eyre by Charlotte Brontë (book)
"Shadows for Silence in the Forests of Hell" by Brandon Sanderson (short story)
Moon Knight (TV series)

YOUR EXAMPLES:

When you are cruel to yourself, contemptuous and shaming, you only increase the cruelty in the world; when you are kind and compassionate toward yourself, you increase the kindness and compassion in the world. Being compassionate toward yourself—not self-indulgent or self-pitying, but kind—is both the least you can do and the single most important thing you can do to make the world a better place. Until you are free, we can't be fully free, which is why all of us together have to collaborate to create that freedom for everyone. Our wellness is tied to yours.

Joyfully Ever After

The stepping stone to joy is feeling like you are "enough," and feeling "not enough" is a form of loneliness. We need other people to tell us that we are enough, not because we don't know it already, but because the act of hearing it from someone else—and (equally) the act of taking the time to remind someone else they're enough—is part of what makes us feel that we're enough. We give and we receive, and we are made whole.

It is a normal, healthy condition of humanity to need other people to remind us that we can trust ourselves, that we can be as tender and compassionate with ourselves as we would be, as our best selves, toward any suffering child. To need help feeling "enough" is not a pathology; it is not "neediness." It's as normal as your need to assure the people you love that they can trust themselves, that they can be as tender and compassionate with themselves as you would be with them. And this exchange, this connection, is the springboard from which we launch into a joyful life.

Wellness, once again, is not a state of mind, but a state of action; it is the freedom to oscillate through the cycles of being human, and this ongoing, mutual exchange of support is the essential action of wellness. It is the flow of givers giving and accepting support, in all its many forms.

The cure for burnout is not self-care; it is all of us caring for one another.

SO, WE'LL SAY IT ONE MORE TIME:

Trust your body.

Be kind to yourself.

You are enough, just as you are right now.

Your joy matters.

Please tell everyone you know.

Please use the following pages for any reflections you've had throughout your work for notes, self-encouragement, whatever you'd like.

How to Practice Mindfulness

Mindfulness has been well studied, with overwhelming evidence to demonstrate how good it is for our well-being. But what is it actually and how do you do it?

There are a lot of different approaches, and this is not meant to be a comprehensive guide to mindfulness—there are many books and courses dedicated to teaching it, if you want to dive into the subject. But if you're working on this book and we use the word "mindfulness" and you're like, "What does that even mean?" here's what we mean.

Mindfulness Is Awareness Without Judgment

It's very easy to drive or cook or almost anything on a kind of "autopilot," where your body is so familiar with the processes and actions that you don't have to be consciously aware of anything you are doing and before you know it, you spent your whole commute thinking about work and suddenly you are home. Mindfulness is the practice of keeping your mind on the task at hand, noticing when your mind starts to wander, and bringing your attention back.

Nonjudgment happens when you pay attention without being distracted by evaluations of how good or bad, pleasant or unpleasant things are.

For example, you notice that your mind is wandering to different thoughts when you were intending to focus on something you were doing. You might automatically scold yourself for letting your mind wander; but a mindful approach would be to **notice that your mind is wandering without labeling it as "bad" or "good," and then just return to what you were intending to focus on.**

A useful practice commonly used as a beginning exercise is **mindful toothbrushing.** It's a thing you're going to do anyway, it only takes a few minutes, and you may as well do it mindfully. So, make the choice to turn your attention to the toothbrushing.

1. **Observe the physical sensations** like touch, taste, and smell. It's easiest to start with sensations directly related to the toothbrushing itself.

2. **Notice any emotional responses you have while brushing your teeth.** Pride in your excellent dental hygiene? Boredom for having to stand in a tiny room

for a few minutes? Maybe you'll notice other internal sensations, like tightness in your neck or shoulder, or clenching in other muscles. **You can choose to release unnecessary tightness or not; all that matters in this exercise is that you noticed it.**

3. **You will almost certainly notice that your mind has wandered,** and your attention has strayed from the present, toothbrushing moment. You'll end up thinking about the past or the future. **And that's great practice because it's an opportunity for you to set those thoughts aside for two minutes while you go back to giving your attention to the toothbrushing.** (2 to 3 min)

Does this sound tedious beyond belief? That's okay because it's only a few minutes! And the research is conclusive about how good it is for you, so remember that it's worth it. (Positive reappraisal FTW!)

While you practice this attention without judgment, your brain is operating in a new way, teaching itself to follow your lead. This lack of judgment is often new to people's brains; judgment is a default response for most of us, and your brain is excellent at accompanying any thought with a spontaneous evaluation. Now your brain is learning to separate the evaluation from the observation. And as your brain wires itself in this new way, it will work its way into other moments in your life.

It might take some time before you notice any difference. That's okay. (Try repeating the practice most days for two months.) The good news is that the more you practice, the easier it gets, broadly speaking. And for a lot of people, the more they do it, the more they like it, and the more they begin applying it to other tasks in their everyday life.

APPENDIX II
How to Listen to Your Body

1. **Start with noticing input from the five senses you were taught about in elementary school: sight, hearing, smell, touch, and taste.** You may notice emotions or memories associated with them. All you have to do is pick a sense and be curious about what that sense has to tell you. Without judging the sensation or your feelings about that sensation, observe it for a few minutes.

You can find mindful eating exercises online, as well as mindful walking guides that usually follow this same procedure. **Do this for a few minutes, most days, for several weeks, or until you discover that you're noticing sensations habitually, without choosing to.**

2. **Next, notice sensations within your own body.** Sight, hearing, smell, touch, and taste all have the job of telling you what's going on outside of your skin. But you also have a sensory system that lets you know what's going on inside your body, which is known as "interoception." This system communicates most readily about acute sensations—your heart racing, your stubbed toe aching, your empty stomach grumbling. Practice noticing these with curiosity, paying attention to the sensations without judging them. You may also notice emotions or memories associated with the sensations. Yoga practices are helpful for this, as they take your body to the edges of its capabilities while your mind is in a quiet state, ready to receive input from your body.

3. **As you do this several times a day for a few weeks, you may find that you can sense more subtle cues.** Maybe you'll notice the need to pee before it's urgent, or that you're dehydrated before you feel thirsty. This is what most people mean when they say, "Listen to your body." You're observing the sensations, and can learn to interpret them, in the most fundamental kind of communication. You're learning your body's language, and it takes time and practice to learn any language.

4. **Now, attend to the intersection of your body and its environment.** Your capacity to perceive how close you are to an object, if you are standing or lying down, or how fast you are moving is called "proprioception." It's a combination of many sensory cues, both inside and outside your body. For example, try standing with your feet together and your arms crossed over your chest. Turn your head slowly from left to right. Now do it again and close your eyes. Lots of folks lose their balance without the visual cue to tell them they are upright. Dancing in a crowd requires you to understand the space between you and others. It usually happens below the level of conscious awareness, but you can practice noticing as your brain takes care of those issues. Listening to proprioception follows the same process as your sense of

external stimuli and your internal experience. Turn your attention toward the motion of your hand as you reach for a pan, and where you place your weight as you chop vegetables.

5. **Practice until your brain can do it without you having to tell it to.** (This might take a few months of regular practice, or a few years of sporadic practice.)

How to Brainstorm

Brainstorming comes naturally to some people, but lots of us could benefit from some guidance. It helps me to think of brainstorming as listening to auditions for chamber choir members.

1. I invite everyone to audition. Every singer/idea is allowed to show up no matter where they come from, no matter what they look like, no matter how unlikely they are to work out. You can never tell until they open their mouth and show you what they've got to offer. Not everyone will sing in the choir, but unless everybody gets a turn, you'll never find the hidden gems.

2. There is a time limit. I can't go on auditioning singers all semester. I have to start rehearsals at some point! Make up whatever duration works for you, but a few minutes is usually enough. Set a timer, then write down everything that comes to mind, ignoring if an idea seems good or bad or silly or random. Don't stop when you get to the first idea you like. Don't try to keep going until you find the "perfect" answer.

3. Thank everyone for showing up, even though most of them won't be singing for you. You needed to discard those possibilities to clear the way for the ones that are going to make the kind of music you're looking for.

4. Go through the list and start identifying the ideas that seem right.

Emily Nagoski, PhD, is the award-winning author of two *New York Times* bestsellers: *Burnout* and *Come as You Are: The Surprising New Science That Will Transform Your Sex Life.* She has an MS in counseling and a PhD in health behavior, both from Indiana University.

Amelia Nagoski, DMA, is the coauthor with her sister, Emily, of the *New York Times* bestselling *Burnout: The Secret to Unlocking the Stress Cycle.* As a conductor and educator, her job is to run around waving her arms while making funny noises and generally doing whatever it takes to help singers get in touch with their internal experience.